Work
Manual
for

Critical
Care
Nursing

A Holistic
Approach

Fourth Edition

Carolyn M. Hudak, R.N., Ph.D.

Adult Nurse Practitioner
Formerly Associate Professor of Nursing and
Assistant Professor of Medicine
University of Colorado Health Sciences Center
Denver, Colorado

Barbara M. Gallo, R.N., M.S.

Assistant Director
Visiting Nurse And Home Care, Inc.
Hartford, Connecticut

Thelma "Skip" Lohr, R.N., M.S.

Instructor, Psychiatric Nursing
Bloomsburg University of Pennsylvania
Bloomsburg, Pennsylvania

Contributing Authors

The authors wish to thank the following people who prepared material for this workbook based
on their contributions to the accompanying text, *Critical Care Nursing: A Holistic Approach,*
fourth edition:

Patricia D. Barry, R.N., M.S.N.
Ann T. Bobal, R.N., B.S.
Patricia K. Brannin, R.N., M.S.N., R.R.T., A.N.P.
Joseph O. Broughton, M.D., F.A.C.C.P.
Helen C. Busby, R.N., B.S.N., C.C.P.
Karen D. Busch, R.N., Ph.D.
Donald E. Butkus, M.D.
Cynthia Johnson Dahlberg, M.A., C.C.C.-Sp.
Frank Davidoff, M.D.
Robert W. Hendee, Jr., M.D.
Shirley J. Hoffman, R.N., B.S.N.
Judith L. Ives, R.N., M.S.
Margaret A. Marcinek, R.N., M.S.N., Ed.D.

Dorothy Murphy Mayer, R.N., B.S.N., C.C.R.N
Naomi Domer Medearis, R.N., M.A., M.B.A.
Joan Mersch, R.N., M.S.
Marilynn Mitchell, R.N., M.S.N., C.C.R.N.
Ann Marie Powers, R.N., M.S.
Suzanne Provenzano, R.N., B.S.N., C.C.R.N., C.N.R.N.
Karen Robbins, R.N., M.S.
William A. Seiffert, M.D.
Julie A. Shinn, R.N., M.A., C.C.R.N.
Janice S. Smith, R.N., M.S.
Rae Nadine Smith, R.N., M.S.
Phillip S. Wolf, M.D.
Sally V. Zouras, R.N., B.S.N.

Work Manual for

Critical Care Nursing

A Holistic Approach

Fourth Edition

J. B. Lippincott Company
Philadelphia
London   New York   Mexico City   St. Louis   São Paulo   Sydney

Fourth Edition

Copyright © 1986, by J. B. Lippincott Company. Copyright
© 1982, 1977, 1973 by J. B. Lippincott Company. All rights
reserved. No part of this book may be used or reproduced in
any manner whatsoever without written permission except in
the case of brief quotations embodied in critical articles and
reviews. Printed in the United States of America. For information address J. B. Lippincott Company, East Washington
Square, Philadelphia PA, 19105.

ISBN 0-397-54590-8

6 5 4 3 2 1

The authors and publisher have exerted every effort to ensure that drug selection and dosage set forth in this text are
in accord with current recommendations and practice at the
time of publication. However, in view of ongoing research,
changes in government regulations, and the constant flow of
information relating to drug therapy and drug reactions, the
reader is urged to check the package insert for each drug for
any change in indications and dosage and for added warn-
ings and precautions. This is particularly important when the
recommended agent is a new or infrequently employed drug.

Preface

This workbook has been compiled in conjunction with the fourth edition of the text, *Critical Care Nursing: A Holistic Approach.* It can be used as an adjunct to the textbook or independently by the student or practitioner who wishes to determine his or her level of comprehension of a specific content area.

This edition of the workbook covers almost all of the content included in the textbook. New to this edition are chapters on cardiovascular diagnostic techniques, cardiac monitoring, percutaneous transluminal coronary angioplasty, autotransfusion, common pulmonary disorders, cerebrovascular disease, and seizure disorders and an innovative chapter on the use of touch as a nursing intervention.

The questions and exercises cover a range of critical care concepts from anatomy and pathophysiology to the emotional aspects of the critical care unit environment. A variety of questioning methods is employed, including questions requiring synthesis and application of knowledge to patient-care situations. Answers follow each set of exercises to provide immediate feedback on performance to the learner.

Material in this workbook can be used as a basis for informal unit inservices, patient-care conferences, and classroom discussions, as an aid in determining the knowledge base of the critical care nurse for orientation purposes, and as a guide for nurses who are preparing for certification examinations.

Carolyn M. Hudak, R.N., Ph.D.
Barbara M. Gallo, R.N., M.S.
Thelma "Skip" Lohr, R.N., M.S.

Contents

Work Manual for

Critical Care Nursing

A Holistic Approach

Fourth Edition

Patient Study Guides

These study guides are offered to help you devise a systematic method for evaluating the status of a patient. As you become more adept at assessment, you will probably develop a method that is "natural" for you. The important principle involves having a logical sequence of assessment that allows you to evaluate all systems when caring for the patient.

Study Guide 1 is intended for use with the patient who is being monitored. It will help you focus on assessing his cardiac status in relation to drug therapy.

Study Guide 2 is a useful tool for patient care conferences or nursing rounds. It suggests a method for focusing discussion on identifying and planning to meet patient care needs and can be helpful in involving other personnel to serve as discussion leaders, as it can be used to outline their preparations.

Study Guide 3 offers another organized method for identifying patient needs. Categories based on broad physiological, sociological, and psychological components are provided along with leading statements to direct the thought process in a specific category.

PATIENT STUDY GUIDE 1

1. What is the rhythm? State your reasons.

2. Drugs received:

3. Responses to drugs:

4. Symptoms:

5. Complications:

6. What are the patient's perceptions and responses to the situation?

PATIENT STUDY GUIDE 2

Suggested Guide for Patient Rounds	Additional Information and Remarks
Purpose	
1. To correlate theory with patients in crisis through small group discussion rather than assigned patient care.	
2. To participate in discussion of nursing judgments with a preceptor.	
Possible approaches to patient selection (you may use one or more)	
1. Major system involved (C-V, renal, CNS, respiratory).	
2. Diagnosis (myocardial infarction, stroke, uremia, emphysema).	

Suggested Guide for Patient Rounds	Additional Information and Remarks
3. Symptoms (chest pain, coma, shock, paralysis). 4. Problem presented to nursing (present complications, may maintain function of other major systems, may be described as nursing diagnoses). You may want to select two patients with the same clinical picture, but different diagnosis, or the same diagnosis, but different clinical pictures for purposes of comparison and individualizing patient care. **Possible approach to planning rounds** 1. Move from familiar, to unfamiliar, back to familiar. Discuss the following: pathology, drugs, other treatments, and nursing care specific for major system involved as well as the support for other systems. 2. Validate, clarify, expand your knowledge with interdisciplinary team members before conference. **Conference** Discuss the information staff will need to know before going to bedside. Direct their thinking to those things that you think are significant (skin color, turgor, edema, respiratory pattern, pulse pressures, behaviors, etc.). Stress major system involved and how it is related to other systems. **At bedside** If possible, allow the staff to ask questions that will gain the information needed, to make observations (listen to chest, take apical pulse, test neuro signs, etc.) that will add to the information, and to engage with the patient, if any treatment is ordered, to become aware of his perceptions. **Follow-up** Discuss observations. You might ask the staff, after they have seen the patient, what nursing care the patient needs. What observations need to be made in the future (for expected, as well as unexpected, complications) to facilitate problem solving? (Example: Patient started on Lasix—check output, CVP, weight, diet replacements, lab studies, ECG changes, skin turgor, etc.)	

PATIENT STUDY GUIDE 3: IDENTIFYING NEEDS OF PATIENTS IN PHYSIOLOGICAL CRISES

Purposes

1. Correlating data pertaining to these needs with knowledge of pathophysiology.

2. Formulating objectives for the planning and giving of expert nursing care.

3. Recognizing the contribution of each staff member to the care of patients in intensive care.

Directions

During patient rounds, identify and note needs of the patients in the space below.

Categories and Descriptions of Nursing Needs

I. PHYSICAL—Needs that are inherent in maintaining a state of physiological homeostasis:

   1. Hygiene, comfort, exercise, rest, etc.

   2. Elements of care that affect the individual's pathologic state—prescribed medication and treatment, for example

II. ENVIRONMENTAL—Needs that stem from the external world and the individual's relationship to it; factors that should be controlled to help the individual adjust to the environment.

III. INSTRUCTIONAL AND INFORMATIONAL—Needs for knowledge that will fortify the patient with a positive attitude that will help him adjust to his return to a normal, yet changed, family and community life.

IV. EMOTIONAL—Needs that stem from his interaction with stressful factors involved with his illness and his ability to cope with stress.

V. COORDINATIONAL—Needs relative to the use of supportive resources and to long-range patient care planning.

   1. Family

   2. Medical and paramedical services

   3. Social services

   4. Community resources

   5. Multidisciplinary team planning for holistic patient care

Stages of Illness: The Patient's Response

STUDY QUESTIONS

1. List the four stages of loss and the major behaviors associated with each stage.

2. What behaviors would lead you to evaluate further whether or not a patient was anxious?

3. In what ways is anxiety similar to other kinds of physiological imbalance such as sodium depletion?

4. How can the nurse enhance a patient's self-esteem?

5. How can the nurse use the theory of grieving and adaptation to illness as a rationale for nursing intervention?

6. What response can the nurse make to a patient's angry, hopeless comment about his disease?

7. This framework describes a patient who maintained denial throughout his hospitalization. Place an *x* where you would talk with him about activity restrictions and give your rationale.

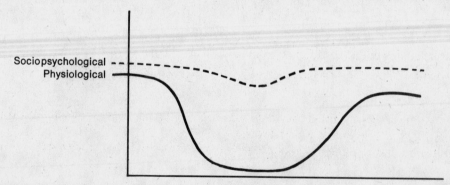

8. This patient had a wide lag both in becoming ill and getting better. The arrow in the diagram indicates when he was transferred from the critical care unit.

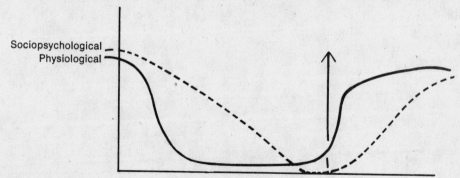

What behaviors would you anticipate at the time of transfer by looking at this pattern?

9. A patient with a long-standing mitral stenosis has had corrective surgery. Using this framework, place an x at the spot where she might show the greatest resistance to taking on more activity, and state your rationale.

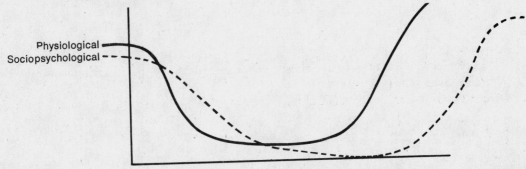

10. A patient with myasthenia gravis has had increasing muscular weakness with two respiratory crises in the past 6 months. She had been working full-time and was independent and realistic about her illness and its limits. During her last hospitalization she seemed less cooperative, harder to please, and more tearful. In terms of this framework, what assumptions can you make about her adaptation to her worsening illness?

11. State whether or not you think the patients described below are ready for an increased amount of learning, and briefly give your reason.
    a) A patient has just been weaned from a respirator and still feels dyspneic.

    b) A patient states that she is feeling good physically and mentally and is looking forward to being transferred out of the critical care unit.

c) A patient recovering from an auto accident is upset upon receiving the news that he has pneumonia and will have to remain in the critical care unit longer.

d) A patient is very reluctant to admit that he has been critically ill.

e) A patient who had been free of chest pain for several days is now receiving medication to ease chest pain.

12. Identify two patient behaviors that you find hard to deal with and the way in which you usually respond or feel.

13. Using the framework in this chapter, plot out the progress of a patient you have recently cared for, based on your observation of his behavior.

14. When should the nurse consider initiating a psychiatric consultation?

15. Each of us experiences anxiety in our lives. The following techniques are designed to lessen anxiety. Try them out on yourself in order to gain experience and confidence before helping a patient or family member use them.

a) Focus on your "self-talk" or internal dialogue. Does it concern a problem that troubles you? Does this dialogue increase your anxiety? Does it contain thoughts that are negative about yourself? If so, say these thoughts out loud to yourself. Think about what you have said and concentrate on changing parts of this self-conversation so that it is more positive and realistic. If, for example, you are worried about an upcoming event, pare the event into bite-sized pieces. Then focus on achieving each one, step by step. Changing what you say to yourself can control anxiety.

b) Try out the following relaxation exercise.

Pick a quiet place where you can lie down.
Take several deep breaths and let them out slowly.
Let your body sink into the couch or mattress so that all body parts are supported.
  Start the muscle tensing and relaxing with your toes and work up toward your head.
  Start by curling your toes as tightly as possible.
  Hold that position for a few seconds and then let go.
  Feel the sensation as your toes unclench.
  Then, point your toes up toward your head as far as possible. You will feel your calf
    muscles tighten.
  Then relax your feet and savor the sensation.
  Next, tighten your thigh muscles by pressing the back of your knees into the couch.
    Hold the position for a few seconds and then relax your knees.
  Continue this process of tensing and relaxing your muscles with your buttocks, abdo-
    men, fingers, upper arms, and shoulders.
Take a few deep breaths and let them out slowly as you go along. Imagine the tension
    draining out of your body as you relax.
As you concentrate on the muscle relaxation, your mind will clear of thoughts.
Before sitting up, enjoy your relaxed feeling for a few moments.

Stages of Illness: The Patient's Response

ANSWERS TO STUDY QUESTIONS

1. Shock and disbelief—denial, lack of cooperation
   Developing awareness—anger, guilt, depression
   Restitution—crying, reminiscing, questioning, expressing fears
   Resolution—overidentification with illness, self-depreciation, recognition of limitations, inter-
   dependence, pride in the accomplished rehabilitation
2. When restlessness, incessant talking, constant or repetitive questioning, joking, glibness or
   flipness or quietness are not part of the patient's everyday behavior, they may indicate anxiety.
   Rising blood pressure, pulse and respirations, dilated pupils, and cool or damp extremities will
   serve as more consistent evidence of anxiety.

3. Each individual seeks to behave in ways that will maintain equilibrium both psychologically and physically. When dehydration occurs, a tension state exists and the individual becomes aware of his thirst. The tension of thirst activates his response of drinking. The fluid lessens the dehydration as well as the thirst, and equilibrium is restored. Anxiety also creates a tension state, and the individual behaves in ways to relieve or lessen the anxiety. For example, a person suddenly becomes seriously ill. The fear arising out of loss of control and the unknown creates tension. One way to reduce this tension is to deny the seriousness of the event. Although this does not solve the problem in the same way that drinking resolves dehydration, it can be an effective way of coping in that it temporarily eliminates the tension.

4. The nurse can enhance the patient's self-esteem by calling him by name and seeking permission when impinging on his hospital space, when sitting on his bed, or opening his bedside stand or drawer; by knocking or announcing her presence before entering his room or curtained space; by providing privacy by closing curtains and draping; by introducing herself and strangers when they come in contact with the patient; by referring questions about the patient to the patient rather than to visitors; and by not talking to others about him in front of him.

5. By understanding both the response to loss and the stages of illness, the nurse can analyze responses and thereby make her communication specific to where the patient is in the process.

6. Any comment that empathizes with feelings about the disease rather than the disease itself is appropriate.

7.

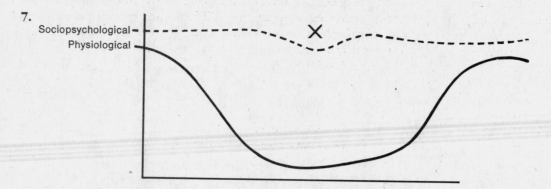

This patient would be most receptive to discussing the necessary changes in his style of living during the slight drop in the dotted line (sociopsychological response). During this time he is slightly more accepting of his illness and may be able to talk more realistically and with less denial about what has happened to him. Teaching on either side of this drop in the dotted line would probably be met with denial—beforehand, because of anxiety, and during convalescence, because the patient is getting better and may feel that there is no need for him to behave any differently than he did before his illness.

8.

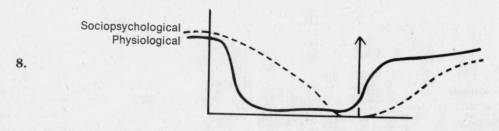

At the time of transfer the patient was physically improving, although his sociopsychological response was lagging and he was still "feeling" ill. Transfer, under these circumstances, will provoke anxiety and regression. The patient may insist that he is not well enough to be moved, he may have many subjective complaints, or his condition may physically worsen. He may backslide to an earlier phase of adaptation and become more dependent, angry, or sad. All of these behaviors indicate that he does not feel ready to cope with the unknown situation that lies ahead.

9.

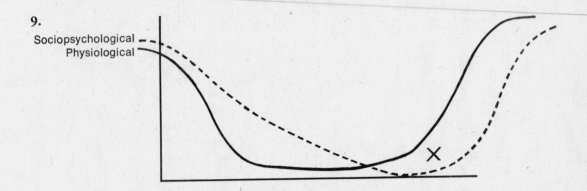

Sociopsychological
Physiological

This patient will resist independence as the lag between her physical and sociopsychological response widens. Although improving physically, she still feels ill. This often occurs when a hospitalization results in better health. Changes in body image, whether they result in limits or in improvement, cause anxiety. Maintaining a former level of dependence will provide comfort until the patient's anxiety lessens. Another reason for maintaining a pre-illness level of adaptation in the face of physical improvement is concerned with secondary gains; that is, ways in which the patient used her illness to have her needs met. Moving to a new level of adaptation when the former pre-illness level was effective also elicits anxiety.

10. This patient had apparently made an effective adaptation to her illness; however, each exacerbation is an additional threat sending her into the cycle of the sick role again. Repeated illness within short periods of time often prevents resolution, and as a result adaptation occurs at an earlier stage. With each exacerbation, the nurse can expect a temporary regression to an earlier level of mastery. At this point in her illness, the patient has behaviors that fit into the stage of developing awareness. She may well be realizing the implications of her deteriorating condition.

11. a) No. Patients struggling to maintain basic physiological functions, such as breathing, usually have little energy left for other activities.

  b) Yes. Learning is likely to occur in quiet stages when the patient's emotional outlook and physical condition correspond.

  c) No. A relapse or movement back on the health-illness continuum is likely to cause anxiety, worry, or depression that will interfere with learning.

  d) No. There is probably a large gap between the patient's physical and emotional outlook if he is experiencing a high degree of denial about the seriousness of his illness. Therefore he will probably be reluctant to learn about facts that reiterate the gravity of his illness.

  e) No. Pain, the effect of pain medication, or worry about the new episode of pain will interfere with the patient's ability to absorb new information.

12. Individualized response
13. Individualized response
14. When the staff feels ill-equipped to deal with the behaviors that the patient is presenting.
    When any one stage of grieving or adaptation seems intractable for a long period of time.
    When the patient's feelings or behaviors are persistently irrational or fail to respond to reality orientation or reality-testing.

When the patient's coping mechanisms are known or observed to be insufficient to handle the trauma. This would include children, already depressed persons, persons who are already in the midst of dealing with a previous loss, and psychotic or severely neurotic persons.

15. **a)** Carry out the exercise as described.
    b) Carry out the exercise as described.

Extending Critical Care Nursing to the Patient's Family

STUDY QUESTIONS

Directions

Respond to the following situations by identifying the feelings the family members are experiencing.

1. The parents of a terminally ill son repeatedly plead to the nurse, "We want the best, no matter what it costs."

   The nurse might say, "You feel . . .

2. A patient is being transferred to a medical unit and the family responds angrily by saying, "She's not ready to be moved. Can't you see that she still has IVs in her?"

   The nurse might say, "You feel . . .

3. The father of a critically burned child cries, "It's all my fault. I left the matches near the lawn mower."

   The nurse might say, "You feel . . .

4. Family members are asked to leave the bedside of a patient, and the family responds bitterly by saying, "You allow the Smiths to stay constantly with their father."

   The nurse might say, "You feel . . .

5. A patient has become disoriented. The family says, "What have you done to him?"

   The nurse might say, "You feel . . .

6. The family repeatedly asks the nurses, "Where is the doctor?"

   The nurse might say, "You feel . . .

7. A distressed patient complains to the family, "I'm being tortured. Get me out of here!" The family looks at the nurse.

   The nurse might say, "You feel . . .

8. The family members continuously advise the nurses regarding small details of patient care. For example, "Yesterday the tube was on her left side and she felt better."

The nurse might say, "You . . .

9. A patient has died after a short but acute illness. Family members become hysterical and accuse the nurses by saying, "Why didn't you take better care of him? Why wasn't someone with him?"

The nurse might say, "You feel . . .

10. The family has just received a very large bill for one week of care in the critical care unit, and they say to the nurse, "How can this be? We have to pay all this money and he doesn't even have a clean gown on when we come to visit!"

The nurse might say, "You feel . . .

11. Briefly describe the nine treatment recommendations for care of the dying patient.

Directions

With your colleagues or classmates, use role playing to enact the following situations until satisfactory solutions are achieved. Take turns and switch roles. Give feedback to one another about the way specific responses made you feel at the moment you heard them. When necessary call in a psychiatric-mental health clinician to help you with communication skills or facilitation.

12. There is little hope that a patient will survive. He must be transferred to a private room in a medical unit in order to make room for a new admission to the critical care unit. The family has

been in the waiting room around the clock for 3 days. The nurse must notify the family of the impending transfer.

13. A nurse returns from her coffee break by way of the waiting room. From the family members of the patients, she learns that someone has arrested and all family members were asked to leave. The families' anxiety appears to be contagious. Some people are pacing while others are talking loudly or crying. Each person seems to believe that it is his relative who is near death. Everyone begins to converge on the nurse asking, "Who has arrested?"

14. A patient has arrested and appears to be dead. There is no physician present at the moment. The family verbally attacks the nurse by saying, "Why didn't you call the doctor? Where is the doctor?"

15. Family members have given up hope for the patient and plead with the nurse to turn off the life-sustaining equipment.

Extending Critical Care Nursing to the Patient's Family

ANSWERS TO STUDY QUESTIONS

1. You feel scared that everything possible is not being done?
2. You feel frightened that she is not ready to be transferred?
3. You feel responsible for the accident?
4. You feel angry that you're being asked to leave now when you really want to stay?

5. You feel frightened by his confusion?

6. You feel concerned that the nurses cannot take care of your father without the doctor?

7. You feel torn about what to do?

8. You really wish you could do more to make her comfortable?

9. You feel hurt and angry that perhaps everything possible was not done?

10. You feel shocked by the large bill, especially when everything seems like it is in such a mess?

11. a) *Competence* is a necessary foundation for giving such care. Technical competence also conveys comfort, reassurance, and concern.

   b) *Concern or compassion* is experienced by the family as care providers become actively involved with them.

   c) *Comfort* is the primary nursing goal for the dying patient. Assuring physical comfort, including pain control, requires constant, judicious decision-making and attention.

   d) *Communication,* especially listening well, will help you discover how each patient deals with his own death.

   e) *Children* are often important people to critically ill patients. When children visit a dying relative, give short, simple explanations that prepare the child and also answer his questions.

   f) *Family cohesion and integration* will help the family through the stress and grief of losing a loved one. Being together and available to support one another is paramount.

   g) *Cheerfulness and a sense of humor* can help a patient and his family relax and behave in their usual ways. This approach requires good timing and sensitivity to the patient's mood.

   h) *Consistency and perseverance* can convey a powerful sense of compassion. Consistency is especially important because complaints and criticism are often directed toward the nurse. Rather than withdrawing, adopt a tolerant, nondefensive attitude.

   i) *Equanimity* includes the capacity to be comfortable with the dying patient and the ability to view the death of a patient as a life-enriching and professionally gratifying experience.

Caring and Touching: Nursing Interventions

STUDY QUESTIONS

Directions

Now that you have an increased understanding of the qualitative symbols of touch behaviors introduced by Weiss, describe how your increased awareness of their effects can have implications on patient care. Identify possible implications for each of the following situations *in relation to the specific qualities of touch identified.*

1. Mrs. G. is an 84-year-old widow who was admitted this morning at 10:00 AM via ambulance. She was found weak and confused lying on her living room floor. It is suspected that she has suffered a stroke.
    a) What are the implications in regard to *intensity* of touch?

    b) What are the implications in regard to the *duration* of touch?

2. Don, an 18-year-old high school athlete, has been in the critical-care unit for six days. Last week he was traumatically injured while working on a new summer job in a factory. His left leg, left foot, and right hand were caught in a large machine. He has had extensive reconstructive surgery and hopes to regain full use of his leg and foot and partial use of his hand.
    a) What are the implications in regard to the *location* of touch?

b) What are the implications in regard to the *frequency* of touch?

3. Mr. A., a 35-year-old businessman, has been admitted to the ICU following a boating accident in which he suffered multiple lacerations and contusions, a mild concussion, and severe fractures of both legs. He is in constant, severe pain and asks for analgesics frequently.
   a) What are the implications in regard to the *sensation* of touch?

   b) What are the implications in regard to the *action* of touch?

4. Briefly identify and describe the major signals of increased need for touch by patients and families in critical-care. Use the letters in the word "touching" as a guide.
   T
   O
   U
   C
   H
   I
   N
   G

Directions

With your classmates, use role-playing to enact the following situations. Make an effort to use touch in a therapeutic and supportive manner in conjunction with effective verbal communication.

5. Mr. J. has been admitted to the ICU with acute pulmonary edema. He is restless, short of breath, and frightened. You are his nurse.

6. You are the charge nurse in the ICU and one of your patients, Mr. B., has just returned from open heart surgery. You are going to bring his wife in to see him for the first time since surgery. You approach her in the waiting room.

7. Mrs. L. has been recovering from a severe episode of gram negative shock. She calls you to her bedside and, weeping, asks, "Am I going to die?"

8. Miss S. is a 90-year-old woman who was transferred to the ICU after an emergency colectomy. She seems to be recovering well from her surgery but has become increasingly confused and disoriented during the evening. After careful evaluation, you suspect sensory deprivation.

Caring and Touching: Nursing Interventions

ANSWERS TO STUDY QUESTIONS

1. a) *Intensity:* Use varying intensities of touch for optimal communication of caring and support. Use both gentle and firm touch.
   b) *Duration:* Consciously allow for moderate to long durations of touch to encourage the patient's fullest integration of the sensory input. This can be even more effective when used with eye contact and verbal interaction.
2. a) *Location:* Don is in a situation in which his body image is a major concern. His being an adolescent makes this an even more sensitive issue. It is important to use touch in a way that sends positive messages about body image and support during this traumatic time. Touching the trunk (giving a backrub and touching his shoulder) may easily convey feelings of caring. Do not avoid touching his injured extremities. Be gentle in order to avoid painful sensations.
   b) *Frequency:* The generous use of touch in your patient care can be a major influence on Don's comfort with his body and on his self-esteem. Frequent use of touch in care is a very powerful mechanism for building other forms of communication as well as for assisting a patient who is fearful and feeling alone.
3. a) *Sensation:* When approaching Mr. A. it may be helpful to remember that touch, when used in a therapeutic way, can help alleviate pain. Be sensitive to the patient's facial expression and his responses to physical contact on different areas of the body. Watch for muscle tension and grimmacing as well as expressions of relaxation and comfort. Talk with the patient and make eye contact when touching him. Avoid pain stimulation when possible, and use touching frequently when it elicits relaxation on the part of the patient.
   b) *Action:* Approach Mr. A without hesitation and yet with a gentle sensitivity to his discomfort. Avoid aggressive and fast movements toward him. Use verbal communication as you approach him, and observe his facial expressions in reaction to your touch.
4. The assessment guide provides a good framework for signals from a patient or family for an increased need for touch.
   T Total amount of touching by family and health care workers is low.
   O Older patient
      Orientation problems
   U Unusual threats to body image or body boundary

C   Consciousness level?
    Communication problems? Intubated? Tracheostomy?
    Crisis situation?
H   High technology at bedside
    High stress period
    Helplessness and hopelessness? Signs of depression
I   ICU psychosis? Confused, restless
N   Normal use of senses?
G   Giving behavior cues? Verbally? Nonverbally?

Patient Responses to the Critical Care Unit

STUDY QUESTIONS

1. What types of normal behavior, used by individuals in a threatening situation, are most patients in crisis units unable to demonstrate?

2. List the five senses involved in considering sensory input.

3. What is unique about the critical care unit environment with regard to both sensory deprivation and sensory overload?

4. Define sensory deprivation.

5. Define sensory overload.

6. List some sources of noise in the crisis care unit that could cause sensory overload.

7. List four symptoms of behavioral changes that may occur in normal adults exposed to periods of sensory deprivation or overload.

8. Would you expect sensory deprivation to have more effect on a normal adult or on a critically ill adult? Justify your answer.

9. What information can a nursing history include that would be helpful in planning care to prevent sensory deprivation or overload?

10. Briefly justify the rationale for using the term *unresponsive* rather than the traditional term *unconscious* for the patient who does not possess motor function.

11. Discuss methods of structuring the environment to offer the opportunity for reality-testing.

12. What is security information? List some examples.

13. List six nursing interventions that can be used in the critical care unit to minimize sensory deprivation and sensory overload.

14. List at least four adverse effects of sleep deprivation.

15. What is periodicity? How can it affect the planning of care in the critical care unit?

16. Discuss methods of encouraging periods of sleep for a patient with orders for vital signs every 4 hours and measurement of urinary output every 2 hours.

17. List and briefly describe five areas of knowledge about the elderly that nurses need to be aware of in order to provide them with optimal care.

Patient Responses to the Critical Care Unit

ANSWERS TO STUDY QUESTIONS

1. Normal defense mechanisms diminished or absent;
   Ability to run from frightening or painful stimuli
   Ability to analyze a situation objectively
   Ability to plan how to control a situation based on objective analysis
2. Visual
   Auditory
   Olfactory
   Tactile
   Gustatory
3. The ability to deprive a patient of meaningful sensory input while exposing him to a continual bombardment of unfamiliar stimuli, causing potential sensory overload.
4. A phenomenon manifested by a variety of symptoms that occurs following a reduction in either the quality or the quantity of sensory input
5. A phenomenon manifested by a variety of symptoms that occurs following an unreasonable increase in the quality or the quantity of sensory input
6. Talking among staff members, cardiac monitors, respirators, telephones, and any machinery such as suctioning units, IPPB machines, addressographs, etc.
7. Loss of sense of time
   Delusions
   Illusions
   Hallucinations
8. Based on information presented in this chapter, a critically ill patient is more vulnerable to the effects of sensory deprivation. He is faced with coping with an illness that demands much of his energy and is not allowed the choice of submitting to sensory deprivation as in an experiment.

The ill patient has no control over the situation and cannot choose to have the situation stopped on demand.

9. This should be highly individualized, but can begin with information regarding a normal 24-hour period of activity, likes and dislikes of sounds (music, TV programs, etc.), normal sleep patterns, job or school, information about the present, and any information that determines what is significant or familiar to the patient.

10. There is no known method of assessing consciousness except when motor response is possible. *Unconscious* carries a connotation of unawareness, and this is not measurable without motion. *Unresponsive* is a label that is measurable and that eliminates the automatic relationship to awareness or lack of it. *Unresponsive* also gives the nurse a meaningful direction to take in planning the patient's care.

11. Include objects such as calendars, clocks, and pictures of familiar objects as a means of reality-testing; discuss where the patient is and the time of day and the month; encourage family and friends to talk to the patient, and assist them with determining information that may be meaningful to the patient.

12. Security information is that information necessary to prevent needless anxiety; it should include both auditory and visual stimuli. Examples include time, place, day, and concrete information that explains, clarifies, and elaborates. Stated another way, it involves telling the patient what, when, who, where, how, and why.

13. Those presented in the chapter are only a beginning and are not intended to limit individual determination of other measures. They include collection of nursing history as a guideline for planning care; placement of a clock within the patient's view; placement of a calendar within the patient's view; vocal explanation of procedures; music; reading from a book on the list of pastime reading; taped messages from a loved one; pictures of children, parents, etc.; placing the patient's favorite picture on the wall; reducing unnecessary noise from machines through planning, and placing noisy machines away from patients.

14. Irritability and anxiety, confusion, hallucinations, physical exhaustion, disruption of metabolic functions (*e.g.*, a change in adrenal hormone production), and even death.

15. It is the occurrence of human functions in a cyclic manner of peaks and troughs. These cycles may be within a 24-hour period or a life cycle of years. It can affect the planning of care in the crisis care unit by preventing unnecessary strain on a patient during periods of low physiological function. It can help in planning periods of undisturbed sleep or rest at physiologically vulnerable times and may some day provide a rationale for drug dosage and the timing of stressful procedures.

16. One way of handling the problem is to use a quantitative drainage bottle and, with the aid of a shielded flashlight, make readings every 2 hours, but drain the container only every 4 hours to lessen the amount of noise and movements in the room. An accurate record can be kept by subtracting the first amount from the second one. Machines that quietly monitor vital signs without disturbing the patient would permit longer periods of sleep as well as observation of vital signs.

17. In order to give optimal care to the elderly, nurses need to have the following knowledge:

    a) *Assess the senses and plan nursing interventions for sensory deficits.* Adequate historical and physical assessment must be made by the nurse to identify the presence and degree of sensory limitations. Diminished vision and hearing are common in the elderly and require compensatory actions by others, such as speaking clearly and in the line of the patient's vision.

    b) *Assess for the symptoms of acute brain syndrome.* Assessing for acute brain syndrome is not always easy, however here are some symptoms which may be present:
        1) Misidentifying people
        2) Memory impairment
        3) Fluctuation in level of awareness
        4) Visual hallucinations
        5) Restlessness, agitation

Try to differentiate between acute and chronic brain syndrome by history taking which includes determining whether the onset was rapid or slow, what the precipitating events were, and what aggravates and what improves the symptoms.

c) *Use of reality orientation as a therapeutic measure*. A rigid, repetitive regimen of giving security information must be adhered to for all patients with orientation problems. Coordination of effort must be present at all times to maintain a firm plan of care.

d) *Apply the concepts of territoriality as it applies to the elderly*. This concept is critical for the elderly in view of historical diminution of their territory at a time when change for them is increasingly difficult. Both the invasion of personal territory and the absence of extensions of territory occur in critical care units; however, both can be minimized by an aware nurse.

e) *Know the views on death and dying commonly held by elderly people*. Listening to the elderly discuss their feelings about dying is essential. Family members and loved ones should also be included in such discussions. The nurse must also confront her own feelings about death and not impose them on the patient.

Cardiovascular Assessment

STUDY QUESTIONS

1. How does bed rest help remedy fluid overload?

2. Why may the patient in heart failure have the following symptoms?
   Oliguria

   Cool limbs

   Fatigue and weakness

   Alteration in cerebration

   Less tolerance to sedatives

3. What is central venous pressure (CVP)? How can it be measured? What may an increase or decrease in the CVP indicate? What affects the accuracy of a CVP reading and why?

4. What is the rationale for "dangling" patients before getting them into a standing position? What helps the nurse decide whether or not a patient is able to progress from dangling to standing?

5. What information can be gathered from a patient by the use of touch?

6. What effect do IPPB and deep breathing have upon the body?

7. What effect does position change have upon the heart?

8. What happens during a Valsalva maneuver and why is it a hazard?

9. Why are symptoms of lung congestion present with (L.) ventricular failure?

10. What parameters would you use to look for signs of (L.) ventricular failure (lung congestion)?

Cardiovascular Assessment

ANSWERS TO STUDY QUESTIONS

1. During bed rest, redistribution and pooling of blood in the liver and extremities occurs, which can reduce plasma volume by 300 to 500 ml. The reduced circulating blood volume decreases the work load of the heart, the heart becomes smaller and more efficient, and cardiac output is increased. Increased cardiac output results in improved renal blood flow, which increases the glomerular filtration rate, and diuresis occurs. This further remedies fluid overload.

2. OLIGURIA: Inefficient pumping action of the failing heart decreases cardiac output and consequently decreases glomerular filtration pressure, and the urinary output drops.
   COOL LIMBS: Reduced cardiac output results in peripheral vasoconstriction as a compensatory mechanism to preserve blood flow to the vital organs.
   FATIGUE AND WEAKNESS: Decreased cardiac output diminishes the oxygen supply to tissues. Anaerobic glycolysis takes place, resulting in an accumulation of lactic acid and an acidotic state.
   ALTERATION IN CEREBRATION: Cerebral cells are very sensitive to the decreased oxygen supply resulting from a reduced cardiac output. Confusion, restlessness, and agitation are signs of cerebral hypoxia.
   LESS TOLERANCE TO SEDATIVES: When liver congestion accompanies heart failure, its metabolic activities are retarded, resulting in slower detoxification of drugs.

3. Central venous pressure is the pressure exerted by the blood in the vena cava or right atrium. It is measured in centimeters or millimeters of water pressure by means of an intravenous catheter positioned in the vena cava or right atrium.

   An increased CVP may indicate fluid overload, congestive heart failure, a vasoconstrictive state, or cardiac tamponade. A decreased CVP may indicate hypovolemia due to blood or fluid loss or vasodilatation.

Accuracy of the CVP reading is affected by the following:

a) *Position*—zero point on the manometer must be level with the patient's right atrium.

b) *Increased interpulmonic pressure*—respirators, deep breathing, or coughing will increase pressure in the great vessels and also cause false-high readings.

c) *Patency of system*—nonpatent system prevents a complete and free fall of the fluid column to equilibrate with the venous pressure.

4. Abrupt change from a prone to sitting or standing position results in hydrostatic effects in blood vessels that tend to decrease blood pressure in the head. This response causes dizziness or loss of consciousness. Gradual position change such as "dangling" allows pressoreceptors located in the thorax and neck to respond to the drop in blood pressure and restore or maintain an adequate pressure.

Assessing parameters indicative of cardiac output will help the nurse determine a patient's readiness to progress in activity. For example, evaluating the patient's sensorium, pulse rate and quality, temperature, and color of extremities will provide information about the heart's ability to cope with the increased activity. Baseline values should be determined prior to beginning activity so that comparisons can be made (*e.g.,* was tachycardia present before the patient's activity was increased?).

5. Pulse quality, rhythm, rate
   Skin temperature
   Skin turgor
   Muscle tension
   Lung expansion
   Thrills

6. Increased pressure within the chest acts as a pump on the great veins. The venous return is increased, and consequently, the cardiac output is also increased. However, in an already compromised heart (such as after myocardial infarction), this rapid influx of blood may lead to cardiac failure.

7. Semi-Fowler's position reduces the radius of the heart and increases the effectiveness of its pumping action. Tidal volume is also improved as gravity pulls the abdominal contents away from the diaphragm and permits better lung expansion; oxygenation of the blood is thus improved. The position of the lower extremities will affect the blood volume; elevating the legs will increase the venous return, while placing them in a dependent position will result in venous pooling and a reduced circulating volume.

8. During a Valsalva maneuver as one "bears down" with the abdominal and perineal muscles, the glottis closes and there is a *tremendous* buildup of intrathoracic pressure. When this pressure is released, there is a great release of blood that flows into the chest and heart forcefully enough to dislodge a plaque or to cause cardiac overload.

9. The buildup of pressure from a failing left ventricle is transmitted in a retrograde fashion to the left atrium, pulmonary veins, and lungs, resulting in symptoms of lung congestion.

10. Breath sounds—for presence of rales
    Character of respirations—rapid, shallow, dyspneic, orthopneic
    Pulse rate—for increases
    Presence of cough
    Heart sounds—for presence of third or fourth sound

Cardiac Auscultation

STUDY QUESTIONS

1. Why is it important for nurses to detect third and fourth heart sounds?

2. What are the characteristics of sound?

3. What produces the majority of the sound when the chest is auscultated?

4. Define systole and diastole.

5. What produces the normal first heart sound?

6. What produces the normal second heart sound?

7. State the location on the chest wall where the following valves are frequently best auscultated: mitral, tricuspid, aortic, and pulmonic.

8. What produces the third heart sound and what is its significance?

9. What produces the fourth heart sound and what is its significance?

10. What is a frequent cause of mitral stenosis, and when in the cardiac cycle does the murmur occur and why?

11. When does the murmur of mitral insufficiency occur and why?

12. When does the murmur of aortic stenosis occur and why?

13. When does the murmur of aortic insufficiency occur and why?

14. Diagram the third and fourth heart sounds and the murmurs.

Cardiac Auscultation

ANSWERS TO STUDY QUESTIONS

1. The nurse should be able to distinguish the protodiastolic, third heart sound from the presystolic, fourth heart sound for the following reasons: There is an estimated 40% mortality rate among patients who develop clinically obvious left ventricular failure. The key diagnostic sign of early congestive heart failure is the development of a third heart sound. The fourth heart sound occurs with systolic overloading notably in hypertension, myocardial infarction, aortic stenosis, pulmonary hypertension, pulmonary stenosis, and cardiomyopathies.

2. Intensity—the force of the amplitude of the vibrations
Pitch—the frequency of the vibrations per unit of time
Duration—the length of time the sound persists
Timbre—the quality dependent upon overtones accompanying the fundamental tone or note

3. The closure of the heart valves produces the majority of the sound.

4. Systole is the time during which the ventricles contract. It begins with the beginning of the first heart sound and ends with the beginning of the second heart sound. Diastole is the time during which the ventricles relax. It begins with the beginning of the second heart sound and ends with the beginning of the next first heart sound.

5. The normal first heart sound is produced by the asynchronous closure of the mitral and tricuspid valves.

6. The normal second heart sound is caused by the closure of the aortic and pulmonic semilunar valves.

7. The mitral valve is frequently best heard at the apex. The tricuspid valve is auscultated at the fifth intercostal space left of the sternum. The aortic valve can be auscultated in the second right intercostal space, and the pulmonic valve is frequently best heard in the second left intercostal space.

8. The third heart sound is caused by the rapid inrush of blood into a nonpliable ventricle. It is one of the first signs in the development of congestive heart failure.

9. The fourth heart sound is believed to be produced by atrial contraction associated with increased resistance to ventricular filling, as in ventricular hypertrophy.

10. A frequent cause is rheumatic heart disease. The murmur occurs in diastole because that is the time when the atria tries to squeeze the volume of blood through the narrowed or stenotic mitral orifice, causing sound production.

11. In the murmur of mitral insufficiency, the pressure in the aorta exceeds the pressure in the ventricle in systole. The blood regurgitates into the ventricle through the incompetent mitral orifice, causing sound production.

12. The murmur of aortic stenosis occurs in systole because the left ventricle is contracting and trying to squeeze the blood through the stenotic aortic valve, causing turbulence of blood flow with resultant sound production.

13. The murmur of aortic insufficiency is heard in diastole. The semilunar valves are incompetent, and blood regurgitates into the ventricle early in diastole while the pressure gradient is greater in the aorta.

14.

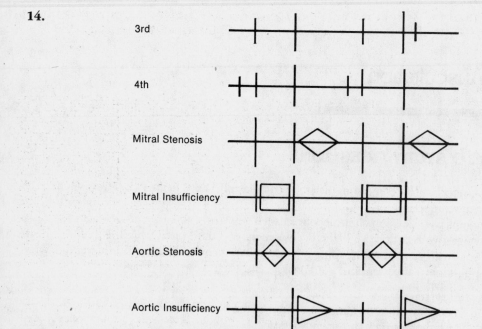

Arrhythmias

STUDY QUESTIONS

Directions

Study each of the following heart tracings, using the questions as a guide. Answer as many of the questions as you can. If you can identify the arrhythmia, write the name above each strip.

1. _____

Rate?_____   P–R interval?_____

P wave rate?_____   QRS interval?_____

R wave rate?_____   T wave configuration?_____

2. _____

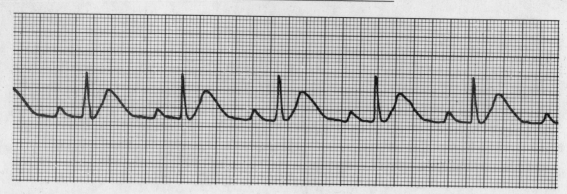

Rate?_____   P–R interval?_____

P wave rate?_____   QRS interval?_____

R wave rate?_____   T wave configuration?_____

3. _____

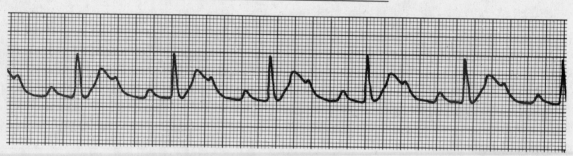

Rate?_____   P–R interval?_____

P wave rate?_____   QRS interval?_____

R wave rate?_____   T wave configuration?_____

4. _____

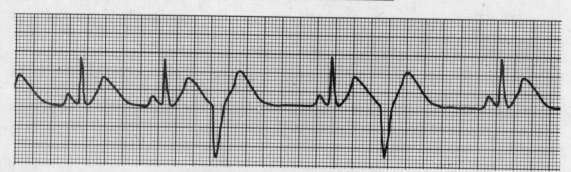

Rate?_____   P–R interval?_____

P wave rate?_____   QRS interval?_____

R wave rate?_____   T wave configuration?_____

5. _____

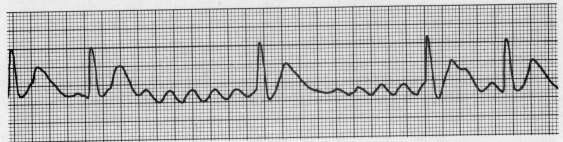

Rate?_____   P–R interval?_____
P wave rate?_____   QRS interval?_____
R wave rate?_____   T wave configuration?_____

6. _____

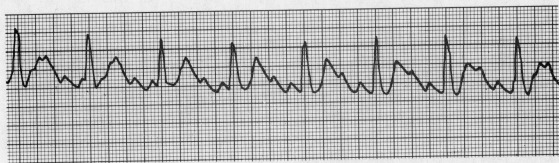

Rate?_____   P–R interval?_____
P wave rate?_____   QRS interval?_____
R wave rate?_____   T wave configuration?_____

7. _____

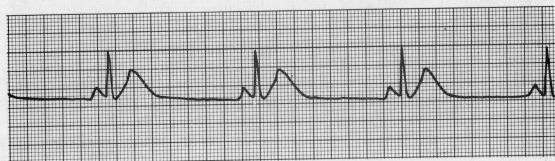

Rate?_____   P–R interval?_____
P wave rate?_____   QRS interval?_____
R wave rate?_____   T wave configuration?_____

8. _____

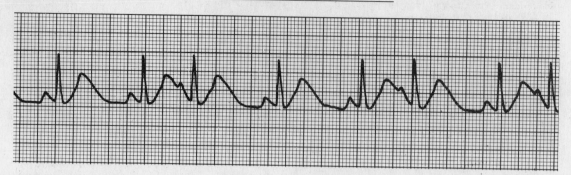

Rate?_____   P–R interval?_____

P wave rate?_____   QRS interval?_____

R wave rate?_____   T wave configuration?_____

9. _____

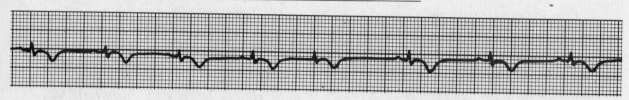

Rate?_____   P–R interval?_____

P wave rate?_____   QRS interval?_____

R wave rate?_____   T wave configuration?_____

10. _____

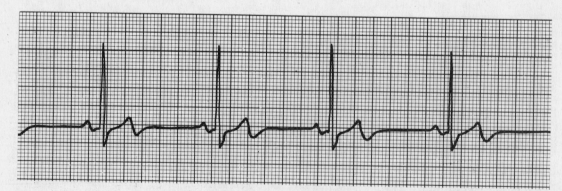

Rate?_____   P–R interval?_____

P wave rate?_____   QRS interval?_____

R wave rate?_____   T wave configuration?_____

11. _____

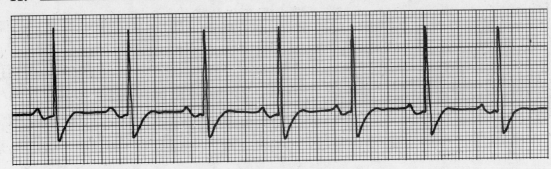

Rate?_____   P–R interval?_____
P wave rate?_____   QRS interval?_____
R wave rate?_____   T wave configuration?_____

12. _____

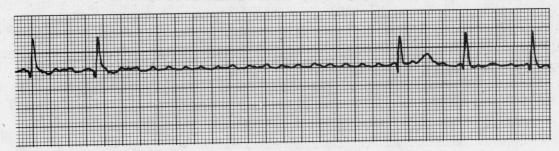

Rate?_____   P–R interval?_____
P wave rate?_____   QRS interval?_____
R wave rate?_____   T wave configuration?_____

13. _____

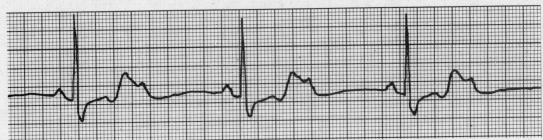

Rate?_____   P–R interval?_____
P wave rate?_____   QRS interval?_____
R wave rate?_____   T wave configuration?_____

14. _____

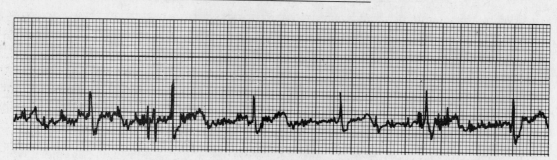

Rate?_____   P–R interval?_____

P wave rate?_____   QRS interval?_____

R wave rate?_____   T wave configuration?_____

15. _____

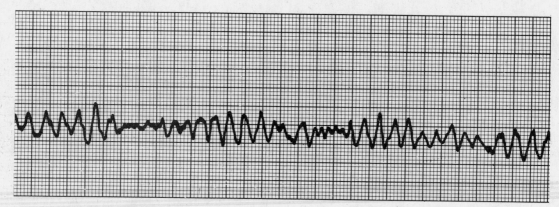

Rate?_____   P–R interval?_____

P wave rate?_____   QRS interval?_____

R wave rate?_____   T wave configuration?_____

16. _____

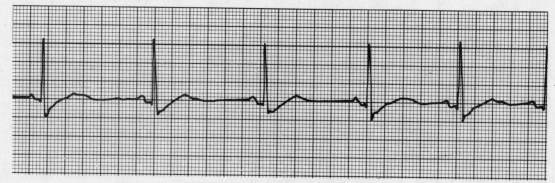

Rate?_____   P–R interval?_____

P wave rate?_____   QRS interval?_____

R wave rate?_____   T wave configuration?_____

17. _____

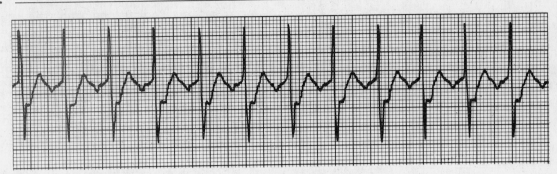

Rate?_____   P–R interval?_____
P wave rate?_____   QRS interval?_____
R wave rate?_____   T wave configuration?_____

18. _____

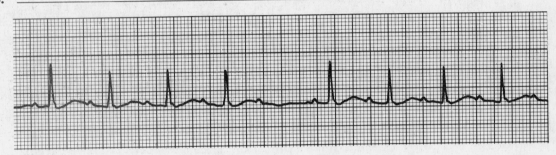

Rate?_____   P–R interval?_____
P wave rate?_____   QRS interval?_____
R wave rate?_____   T wave configuration?_____

19. _____

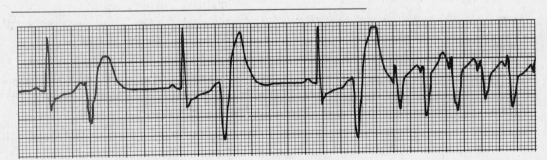

Rate?_____   P–R interval?_____
P wave rate?_____   QRS interval?_____
R wave rate?_____   T wave configuration?_____

20. _____

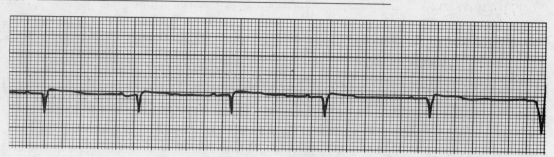

Rate?_____ P–R interval?_____

P wave rate?_____ QRS interval?_____

R wave rate?_____ T wave configuration?_____

21. _____

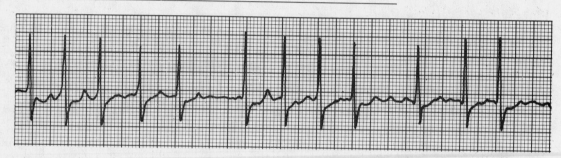

Rate?_____ P–R interval?_____

P wave rate?_____ QRS interval?_____

R wave rate?_____ T wave configuration?_____

22. _____

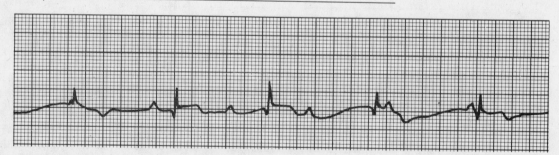

Rate?_____ P–R interval?_____

P wave rate?_____ QRS interval?_____

R wave rate?_____ T wave configuration?_____

Arrhythmias

ANSWERS TO STUDY QUESTIONS

1. Ventricular fibrillation
2. First degree heart block
3. 2 : 1 heart block
4. Ventricular bigeminal beats (VPCs)—unifocal
5. Atrial flutter and fibrillation
6. Atrial flutter with 3 : 1 block
7. Sinus bradycardia
8. Premature atrial contractions (APCs)
9. Premature junctional contraction (PJC), 5th complex
10. Bradycardia
11. Normal sinus rhythm
12. Atrial flutter with high degree of block due to digitalis
13. Second degree block
14. Artifact—loose leads
15. Ventricular fibrillation
16. Sinus arrhythmia
17. Nodal tachycardia—P waves upside down; precede QRS
18. Wenckebach
19. Bigeminal VPCs—VPC hit on top of T wave and into ventricular tachycardia
20. Bradycardia
21. Atrial fibrillation with rapid ventricular response
22. Complete third degree block

Cardiovascular Diagnostic Techniques

STUDY QUESTIONS

1. "Hot-spot" technetium scanning would be indicated in which of the following?
   a) A patient who presented to the emergency room 2 hours after development of symptoms of crushing chest pain
   b) A patient who presented to the anesthesia induction room preoperatively with ECG changes showing new ST segment elevation in the inferior leads
   c) A patient who develops a left bundle branch block pattern on the ECG 2 hours after coronary artery bypass grafting
   d) A patient 10 days post–myocardial infarction who develops angina while showering

2. Long-term ambulatory monitoring is indicated in a patient with which of the following?
   a) Symptoms of dizziness and syncope
   b) The new onset of exertional angina
   c) A right bundle branch block on the ECG
   d) Unstable angina

3. Thallium scanning:
   a) is used in conjunction with an exercise test to evaluate ventricular wall motion
   b) is also known as "hot-spot" imaging
   c) is done in the cardiac catheterization laboratory
   d) is used in conjunction with an exercise test to evaluate myocardial perfusion

4. The diagnostic procedure that is used to evaluate and treat life-threatening arrhythmias is:
   a) nuclear magnetic resonance
   b) phonocardiography
   c) cardiac catheterization
   d) electrophysiology testing

5. Nursing care in the period immediately following cardiac catheterization and coronary arteriography includes which of the following?
   a) Checking pulses in the unaffected limb
   b) Strict fluid restriction
   c) Frequent vital sign assessment for the first several hours
   d) Unrestricted patient activity

Cardiovascular Diagnostic Techniques

ANSWERS TO STUDY QUESTIONS

1. c
2. a
3. d
4. d
5. c

Serum Electrolyte Abnormalities and the Electrocardiogram and Serum Enzyme Studies

STUDY QUESTIONS

1. What are the electrocardiographic indications of hypokalemia and hyperkalemia?

2. Which electrolyte imbalance and which drug effects may be indicated by a shortened Q–T interval? By a prolonged Q–T interval?

3. What is an enzyme?

4. What is the cause for certain enzyme elevations in the serum after acute myocardial infarction?

5. Name the three cardiac enzymes most commonly used in the diagnosis of acute myocardial infarction. Which is the first to rise and which is the last?

6. The following patients have been admitted to your critical care unit with the diagnosis of possible acute myocardial infarction. Discuss the diagnostic value of serum enzyme studies in each situation.
   a) A 36-year-old man who developed chest pain while skiing 6 hours ago.

   b) A 60-year-old chronic alcoholic with progressively increasing symptoms of indigestion over the past 4 days.

   c) A 46-year-old man admitted 12 hours ago to a medical unit with nausea, vomiting, and stomach pains. He received four intramuscular injections of an antiemetic and two intramuscular injections of a narcotic.

d) A 67-year-old woman who developed chest pain while visiting her husband in the hospital 30 minutes ago.

e) A 54-year-old-man with a continuously functioning implanted pacemaker and with chest discomfort for the past 24 hours.

Serum Electrolyte Abnormalities and the Electrocardiogram and Serum Enzyme Studies

ANSWERS TO STUDY QUESTIONS

1. Hypokalemia may be manifested on the electrocardiogram by the development or increased height of the U wave, flattening and inversion of the T wave, ST segment depression, and ultimately by arrhythmias. Hyperkalemia may be indicated by tall, narrow, peaked T waves; signs of intra-atrial, A–V nodal, and intraventricular block; and ultimately ventricular fibrillation.

2. A shortened Q–T interval may indicate hypercalcemia or digitalis effect. Lengthening of the Q–T interval may be caused by hypocalcemia or by quinidine or procainamide (Pronestyl).

3. An enzyme is a protein found in all living cells. Its function is to accelerate the rate of chemical reactions.

4. Serum elevation of cardiac enzymes occurs as the result of necrosis of myocardial cells that contain these enzymes. The damaged cells release their enzymes into the bloodstream.

5. The three cardiac enzymes most commonly used in the diagnosis of acute myocardial infarction are CPK, which rises and falls first; SGOT; and LDH, which rises and falls last.

6. **a)** The 36-year-old man who developed chest pain 6 hours ago while skiing may have some serum elevation of CPK because of strenuous physical exertion. In order to rule out acute myocardial infarction, CPK isoenzymes will be required to differentiate muscle tissue and cardiac tissue as the source. Since LDH elevation does not occur until 12 to 24 hours after myocardial infarction, this enzyme will probably not be elevated. SGOT may be starting to elevate at 6 hours after symptom occurrence, but this is a very nonspecific enzyme with a very widespread distribution, including skeletal muscle tissue, and would probably have already risen because of physical exertion.

   b) The 60-year-old chronic alcoholic with indigestion over the past 4 days will probably have chronic SGOT and LDH elevation because of liver insult. LDH isoenzymes may help to determine whether any of the total LDH elevation is due to cardiac damage if the cardiac fraction of the LDH has not returned to normal by now. If he did sustain an acute myocardial infarction 4 days ago, an elevated CPK would probably have returned to normal by now. None of the cardiac enzymes would be very helpful in diagnosing myocardial infarction, and one would have to rely on the ECG and clinical symptomatology to make the diagnosis.

c) The 46-year-old man admitted 12 hours ago who received intramuscular injections for nausea and stomach pain may have some elevation in SGOT because of muscle trauma caused by the injections; however, if it is massively elevated, one can suspect myocardial infarction. If infarction has occurred, serum CPK will be elevated because of the infarction and because of the injections. For this reason, CPK isoenzymes may help to determine how much of the elevation is due to cardiac tissue release of the enzyme. At 12 hours after onset of symptoms, the LDH elevation may not yet have begun.

d) The diagnosis of the 67-year-old woman who developed chest pain while visiting her husband in the hospital 30 minutes ago will not be aided by serum enzymes. It is too soon for any of the enzymes to have begun rising, and the battery of laboratory tests will have been wasted. She may also have a normal ECG at this point. One cannot rule out acute myocardial infarction until the diagnosis can be more definitely made by enzyme elevations and ECG changes.

e) The 54-year-old man with a pacemaker and 24 hours of symptoms is the perfect candidate for the entire gamut of enzyme tests. At 24 hours after symptom occurrence all three enzymes have probably begun rising, and none would have returned to normal yet. A history should carefully be taken to rule out other causes for enzyme elevation. The pacemaker will preclude any ECG changes that might have aided in the diagnosis of myocardial infarction. Diagnosis will rest solely on clinical symptoms and serum enzyme elevations.

Hemodynamic Pressures

STUDY QUESTIONS

1. Pressure = _____ × _____
2. Normal pressure values for the following are:

$\overline{RA}$	_____torr	$\overline{PAW}$	_____torr
RV systole	_____torr	LA	_____torr
RV end diastole	_____torr	LV systole	_____torr
PA systole	_____torr	LV end diastole	_____torr
PA diastole	_____torr	Ao systole	_____torr
$\overline{PA}$	_____torr	Ao diastole	_____torr
		Ao or MAP	_____torr

3. Identify the systolic and diastolic phases of the left ventricular wave-form.
   a) Aortic valve closure
   b) End diastole
   c) Passive atrial filling
   d) Isovolumetric contraction
   e) Atrial systole
   f) Aortic valve opens
   g) Maximum ejection

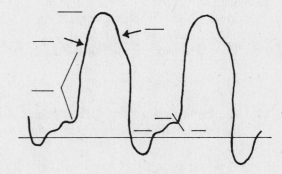

4. On the RA pressure tracing, the:
   a) *a* wave represents _____atrial diastole
   b) *c* wave represents _____atrial systole
   c) *v* wave represents _____bulging of the closed tricuspid valve into the RA
5. On the PA tracing, the dicrotic notch represents (opening, closure) of the (pulmonic, aortic) valve.
6. On the Ao tracing, the dicrotic notch represents (opening, closure) of the (pulmonic, aortic) valve.
7. Right ventricular isovolumetric contraction ends with the opening of the _____ valve.
8. Left ventricular isovolumetric contraction ends with the opening of the _____ valve.

9. The PAW pressure is significant because it reflects left ventricular function. Complete the following formula.

$$PAd \approx \underline{\hspace{2cm}}$$
$$\underline{\hspace{2cm}} \approx \underline{\hspace{2cm}}$$
$$\underline{\hspace{2cm}} \approx \underline{\hspace{2cm}}$$

10. The PAW pressure tracing has two positive waves, the *a* wave and the *v* wave. Match the following.

The *a* wave corresponds with:

_____

_____

_____

_____

a) LA diastole
b) LV systole
c) opened mitral valve
d) LVEDP
e) LA systole
f) LV diastole
g) closed mitral valve

The *v* wave corresponds with:

_____

_____

_____

11. Match the following:
   a) Tricuspid stenosis would elevate the _____.
   b) Tricuspid insufficiency would elevate the _____.
   c) Pulmonary stenosis would elevate _____.
   d) Pulmonary insufficiency would elevate the _____ pressure tracing.
   e) Hypervolemia would elevate the _____.
   f) Mitral stenosis would elevate the _____.
   g) Mitral insufficiency would elevate the _____.
   h) Aortic stenosis would elevate the _____.
   i) Aortic insufficiency would elevate the _____.

   1) LA *v*-wave pressure
   2) RV systolic pressure
   3) LVEDP
   4) RA *a*-wave pressure
   5) LA *a*-wave pressure
   6) RV end-diastolic pressure
   7) RA *v*-wave pressure
   8) RA pressure
   9) LV systolic pressure

12. Match the following:
   a) RV failure would elevate _____.
   b) LV failure would elevate _____.
   c) Pulmonary hypertension would elevate _____.
   d) Constrictive pericarditis or cardiac tamponade would elevate _____.

   1) PAW
   2) Diastolic pressure in all chambers
   3) RV, RA, and systemic pressures
   4) PA, RV, RA

13. The nurse working with the patient whose PAW pressures are steadily increasing knows that the patient's heart failure is (improving, deteriorating).

14. In order to prevent complications in the patient with invasive monitoring, the nurse will:
   a) have the patient do exercises or perform passive exercises for the patient.
   b) cleanse the catheter insertion site and observe for signs of inflammation.
   c) instruct the patient in deep-breathing exercises.
   d) encourage the patient to change positions between pressure measurements.
   e) all of the above

15. The nurse working with the patient notes the following on the oscilloscope:

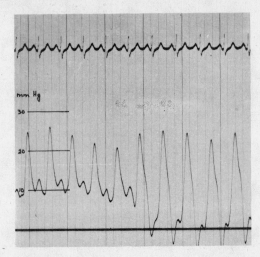

She knows immediately that:
Circle appropriate answer(s)

a) The PAd has decreased.

b) There is nothing to be concerned about, but she will tell the physician when he visits the patient.

c) One of the stopcocks must be open from the transducer to atmospheric pressure.

d) The catheter has floated from the PA into the RV.

e) There is catheter fling in the line.

16. Identify the following normal pressure tracings.

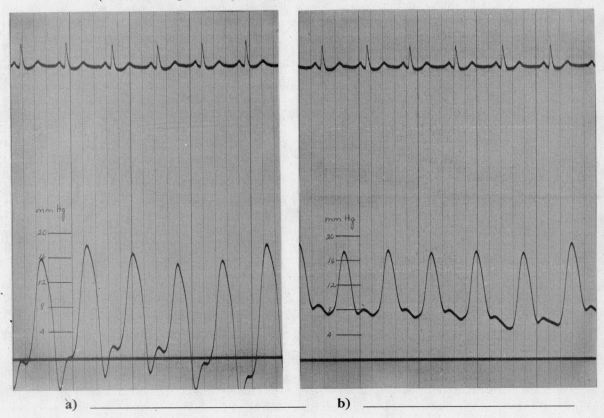

a) _____   b) _____

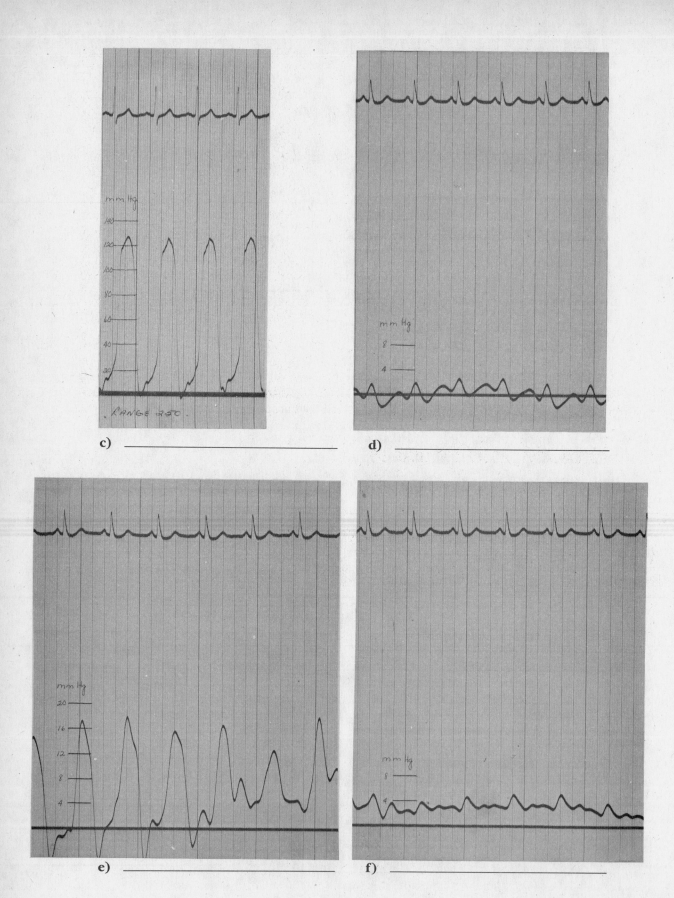

c) _____

d) _____

e) _____

f) _____

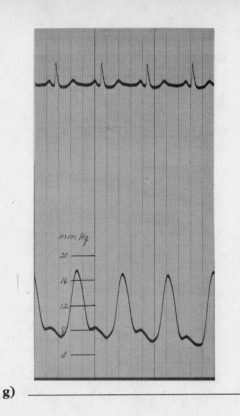

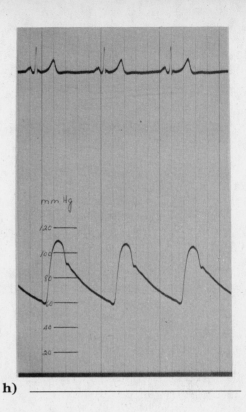

g) _____

h) _____

Hemodynamic Pressures

ANSWERS TO STUDY QUESTIONS

1. flow × resistance

2.

< 6 torr	< 12 torr
<30 torr	< 12 torr
< 5 torr	<140 torr
<30 torr	< 12 torr
<10 torr	<140 torr
<20 torr	< 90 torr
	70–90 torr

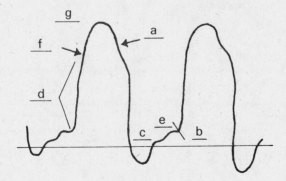

4. **c**
   a
   b
5. closure; pulmonic
6. closure; aortic
7. pulmonic
8. aortic
9. $\overline{PAd} \approx \overline{PAW}$
   $\overline{PAW} \approx \overline{LA}$
   $\overline{LA} \approx LVEDP$
10. c   a
    d   b
    e   g
    f
11. **a)** 4
    b) 7
    c) 2
    d) 6
    e) 8
    f) 5
    g) 1
    h) 9
    i) 3
12. **a)** 3
    b) 1
    c) 4
    d) 2
13. deteriorating
14. **e**
15. **d**
16. **a)** Right ventricular tracing
    b) Pulmonary artery tracing
    c) Left ventricular tracing
    d) Right atrial tracing
    e) Right ventricular to pulmonary artery tracing
    f) Pulmonary artery wedge tracing
    g) Pulmonary artery tracing
    h) Aortic tracing

Cardiac Output

STUDY QUESTIONS

1. Define cardiac output.

2. Define cardiac index.

3. Name two conditions that result in decreased venous return to the right side of the heart.

4. Name two disease states that result in abnormally high cardiac output.

5. The thermodilution method of determining cardiac output is based on which of the following:
   a) Dye concentration
   b) Blood temperature change
   c) Pulmonary oxygen consumption

6. It is important to use the proper computation constant because it allows the computer to account for the _____ and _____ of the injectate that is being used.

7. Optimal cardiac output determinations are obtained using _____ ml of 5% dextrose in water at _____ temperature and injected in not more than _____ seconds.

8. List two possible complications that must be watched for immediately after injection of the cold solution.

9. The cold solution is injected through the _____ lumen of the Swan-Ganz catheter into the _____ chamber of the heart.

10. List five measures that must be used to maintain electrical safety for the patient who has a Swan-Ganz thermodilution catheter.

11. The patient who has cardiogenic shock can be expected to have a (high, low) mean arterial pressure, (high, low) cardiac output and cardiac index, (high, low) pulmonary capillary wedge pressure, (high, low) pulmonary artery diastolic pressure, and (high, low) systemic vascular resistance.

12. The above hemodynamic parameters in the patient with cardiogenic shock indicate the need for treatment with _____ and _____.

13. The patient with septic shock can be expected to have a (high, low) mean arterial pressure, (high, low) cardiac output and index, and (high, low) systemic vascular resistance.

14. If one hemodynamic parameter measurement does not correlate with other parameters and the patient's clinical status, the critical care nurse should:
    a) _____
    b) _____

Cardiac Output

ANSWERS TO STUDY QUESTIONS

1. Cardiac output is the amount of blood that is pumped out of the heart expressed in liters per minute.
2. Cardiac index is cardiac output relative to body surface area, or cardiac output divided by the body surface area.
3. Severe hemorrhage, dehydration, PEEP
4. Septic shock, beriberi, thyrotoxicosis, fever, certain tumors
5. b
6. volume; temperature
7. 10; 0°–40°C; 4
8. Cardiac arrhythmias and migration of catheter to wedge position or into right ventricle
9. proximal; right atrial

10. Nonelectric bed; change wet linens; use of minimal electrical equipment that is well-grounded; inspect computer cable; cap thermistry "tail"; cable not connected to catheter during insertion; use battery power; no simultaneous contact between catheter or patient and other electrical equipment; dry and clean computer and cable; no explosive anesthetic agents

11. low; low; high; high; high

12. addition of volume; vasodilators

13. low; high; low

14. **a)** troubleshoot equipment.

     b) repeat measurements.

Cardiac Monitoring

STUDY QUESTIONS

1. In the standard limb leads, the left leg electrode is always (positive, negative) and the right arm electrode is always (positive, negative).
2. Right and left bundle branch blocks are most easily differentiated on the monitor in lead (II, MCL_1).
3. Ventricular ectopy is most easily differentiated from supraventricular ectopy in lead (II, MCL_1).
4. Acute myocardial infarction can be accurately diagnosed on the cardiac monitor.

          TRUE   FALSE

5. The monitor alarm should be turned off when excessive artifact is present in order to avoid disturbing the patient.

          TRUE   FALSE

6. The monitor technician should never be assigned to additional tasks while he is responsible for monitor observation.

          TRUE   FALSE

Cardiac Monitoring

ANSWERS TO STUDY QUESTIONS

1. positive; negative
2. MCL_1
3. MCL_1
4. False. The cardiac monitor is used for arrhythmia diagnosis. A twelve-lead ECG is necessary for diagnosis of acute myocardial infarction.
5. False. The alarm should only be turned off for short periods of time while electrodes are being changed or for physical care when the nurse is with the patient.
6. True. The observer's attention should not be distracted from the monitors.

Artificial Cardiac Pacing

STUDY QUESTIONS

1. The transvenous endocardial pacemaker is placed in the (right, left) side of the heart and will produce a (positive, negative) paced QRS in the modified V_1 lead.

2. The pacing electrode in the bipolar catheter is the (positive, negative) electrode at the tip of the catheter, and the sensing electrode is the (positive, negative) electrode proximal to the catheter tip.

3. The VVI pacemaker is:
   a) AV sequential
   b) ventricular demand
   c) ventricular fixed-rate
   d) atrial demand

4. The DDD pacemaker is capable of pacing (the atrium, the ventricle, both chambers) and sensing in (the atrium, the ventricle, both chambers).

5. Complete heart block is always an indication for pacemaker insertion.

TRUE   FALSE

6. Pacing catheter perforation of the ventricular wall almost always causes cardiac tamponade and should always be considered an emergency.

TRUE   FALSE

7. Patients who have permanent pacemakers must sell their microwave ovens and electric shavers.

TRUE   FALSE

8. Not all patients are ready to accept information about living with a pacemaker immediately after insertion.

TRUE   FALSE

9. Considering the amount of information about pacemakers that is available to the public, the nurse may assume that the patient already has some knowledge about basic pacemaker function.

TRUE   FALSE

10. Pacemakers impose very few limitations on the patient once he has recovered from the permanent pacemaker insertion procedure.

    TRUE   FALSE

11. The VOO pacemaker is inhibited by a ventricular ectopic beat.

    TRUE   FALSE

12. The VVI pacemaker is inhibited by a ventricular ectopic beat.

    TRUE   FALSE

13. Which of the two types of second degree block is most likely to require pacing: Mobitz I or Mobitz II? Why?

14. What is the advantage of AV sequential pacing over ventricular pacing?

15. Why are pacing and sensing thresholds measured for permanent pacemakers?

16. List three electrical safety precautions that should be adhered to for the temporary pacemaker patient.

17. List three possible symptoms of pacemaker malfunction that should be discussed with the patient.

18. Which of the following cardiac monitor strips indicates improper function of the temporary demand VVI pacemaker? Why? What actions can be taken to correct each problem?

a

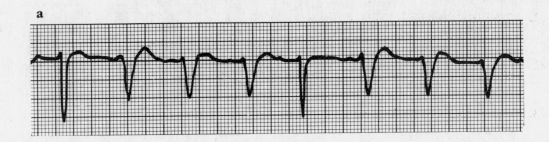

b

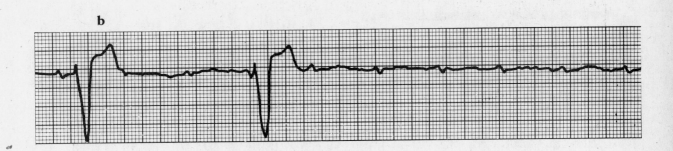

c

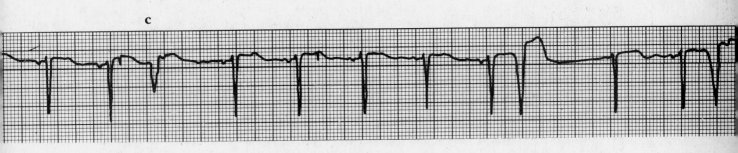

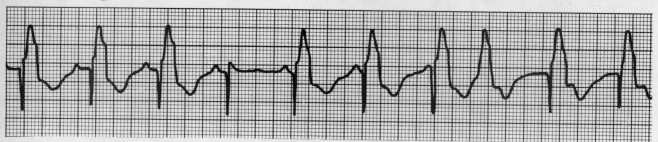

d

Artificial Cardiac Pacing

ANSWERS TO STUDY QUESTIONS

1. right; negative
2. negative; positive
3. **b** Pacing and sensing occur in the ventricle, and pacing is inhibited by spontaneous ventricular electrical activity.
4. both chambers; both chambers
5. False. It is not if the patient has a junctional rhythm with an adequate rate, and the cause of the block is transient.
6. False. Perforation *can* result in cardiac tamponade, but does so infrequently; however, the blood pressure should be checked at frequent intervals after perforation. Remember that the pacemaker patient may not be able to increase his effective heart rate to compensate for a drop in blood pressure. If the patient has underlying AV block, the sinus node rate may increase in an attempt to compensate, but without ventricular response.
7. False. Microwaves and small appliances do not affect pacemakers that are in current use.
8. True. They may not retain this information until they have accepted the pacemaker as a fact of life.
9. False. Don't assume *anything*!
10. True.
11. False. The VOO pacemaker paces the ventricle but has no sensing capabilities. It is a fixed-rate ventricular pacemaker.
12. True. The VVI pacemaker paces the ventricle and has a sensing electrode in the ventricle. It is a ventricular demand pacemaker.
13. Mobitz II, because it results in a less stable rhythm and may result in complete block with an inadequate rate or ventricular standstill.
14. Atrial and ventricular contraction in proper sequence results in higher stroke volume and more optimum hemodynamics.
15. They are measured to obtain electrode placement that will result in consistent pacing without high levels of energy output and sensitivity in the generator, thus prolonging battery life.

16. Nonelectric bed; tap bell instead of electric call light; battery-operated appliances; no simultaneous contact of patient and electrical equipment; minimal amount of electrical equipment, and that present should be properly grounded; dry linens

17. Dizziness, fainting, chest pain, shortness of breath, undue fatigue, fluid retention

18.   **a)**   Properly functioning demand pacemaker. Stimulus discharge is appropriate and each "spike" is followed by a QRS, indicating ventricular capture. The first and fifth complexes are the patient's spontaneous beats and are sensed by the pacemaker and inhibit it.

   b)   This strip demonstrates periods of nondischarge by the pacemaker, as indicated by the absence of pacing spikes. The nurse should check connections at the generator terminals, replace generator batteries, replace generator, and convert to a unipolar system. If these efforts fail to restore pacing, the pacing lead should be replaced. In the meantime, cardiopulmonary resuscitation may be indicated.

   c)   A malfunctioning pacemaker is evident in this strip because of inappropriate sensing. Pacing spikes are noted that should have been inhibited by the previous spontaneous QRSs. Ventricular capture occurs after the last two spikes. One would not expect capture by the first two artifacts because they occur during the refractory period of the preceding QRS. The nurse should increase the sensitivity of the generator, reposition the patient, replace generator batteries, turn pacemaker off if it discharges on the vulnerable phase of the T wave, and notify the physician. The pacing lead may need to be replaced.

   d)   Noncapture is indicated in this strip because of a pacing artifact that is not followed by a QRS. The nurse should increase the MA on the generator, reposition the patient, replace batteries or generator, and administer appropriate drugs or cardiopulmonary resuscitation if frequent or continuous noncapture causes the patient to become symptomatic.

Cardiovascular Drugs

STUDY QUESTIONS

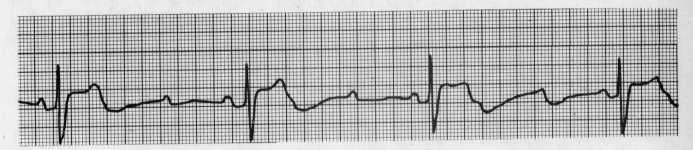

1. A patient with a history of an acute inferior myocardial infarction has an ECG showing the above rhythm. He is also having pain. Which one of the following would you give?

   a) Morphine
   b) Morphine and atropine
   c) O_2
   d) Valium

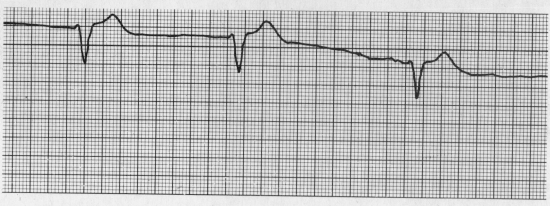

2. A man, age 56, was admitted with severe congestive heart failure. He was given 2.0 mg of digoxin IV with the resulting rhythm. Appropriate R$_x$ now should include *one* of the following:

    a) 0.25 mg digoxin IV
    b) 10 mg KCl IV
    c) Transvenous pacemaker
    d) 1 ampul CaCl$_2$ IV

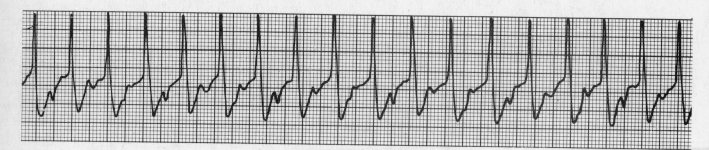

3. The above arrhythmia could result from which *one* of the following?

    a) 100-mg bolus of lidocaine IV
    b) Rapid infusion of isoproterenol (Isuprel)
    c) Excessive sedation with diazepam (Valium)
    d) IV propranolol (Inderal)

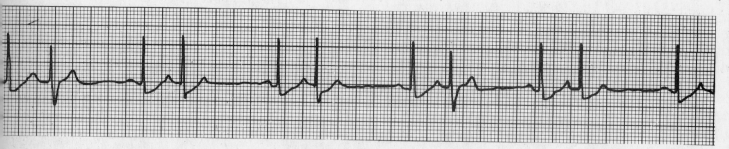

4. The above arrhythmia was observed in a female, age 45. Proper R$_x$ might include *any except one* of the following:

    a) Digoxin
    b) Quinidine
    c) Propranolol (Inderal)
    d) Epinephrine

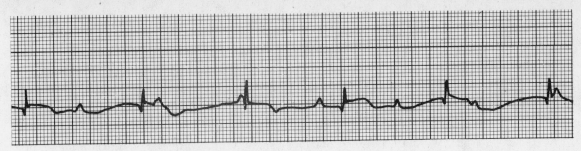

5. Proper R$_x$ of the above arrhythmia might include *all but one* of the following:

    a) IV procainamide (Pronestyl)
    b) Isoproterenol (Isuprel)
    c) Discontinuation of lidocaine drip
    d) Transvenous pacemaker

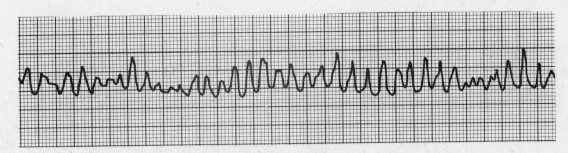

6. If a nurse encounters this rhythm, proper action is to:

    a) telephone the operator.
    b) initiate artificial respiration.
    c) check BP.
    d) provide immediate defibrillation.

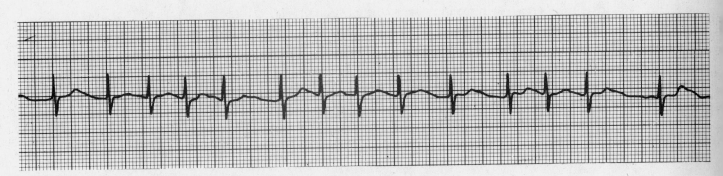

7. A patient on no medication is admitted with the above arrhythmia. The drug of choice is:

    a) Lidocaine
    b) Digoxin
    c) Isoproterenol (Isuprel)
    d) IV quinidine

8. If drug R$_X$ of the previous rhythm is unsuccessful, another accepted method of treatment could be:

   a) Pacing
   b) Cardioversion
   c) Heart lung bypass
   d) Mitral commissurotomy

9. This patient was started on procainamide (Pronestyl) 500 mg q6h. Two weeks later she developed signs of Pronestyl toxicity. She might show *all but which one* of the following set of symptoms:

   a) Fainting
   b) Fever, skin rash, and arthritis
   c) Positive L.E. cell preps
   d) Yellow vision

10. Ideally, procainamide (Pronestyl) should be administered according to:

    a) Pronestyl blood levels
    b) A "q6h" schedule
    c) Body weight
    d) Size of infarct

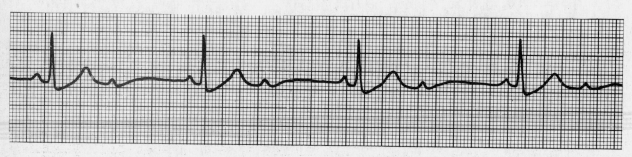

11. This rhythm is important for *all* but *one* of the following reasons:

    a) It may progress to complete heart block.
    b) It should be treated with digitalis.
    c) It will ordinarily respond to isoproterenol (Isuprel).
    d) A transvenous pacemaker should be inserted if the patient has had a myocardial infarction.

12. A patient with a 4 mg/ml drip of lidocaine running rapidly may show which *one* of the following signs:

    a) Fever
    b) Diarrhea
    c) Grand mal seizures
    d) Acute gout

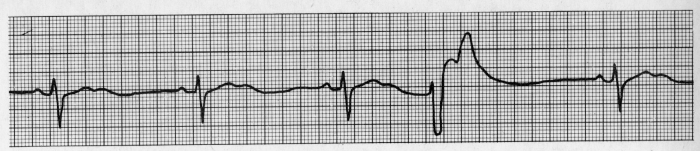

13. A patient with the above rhythm would be treated with which *one* of the following?

   a) Lidocaine
   b) Atropine
   c) Digoxin
   d) Pacemaker

14. Which of the following drugs *decreases* the contractility of the heart muscle?

   a) Digitalis
   b) Glucagon
   c) Propranolol (Inderal)
   d) $CaCl_2$

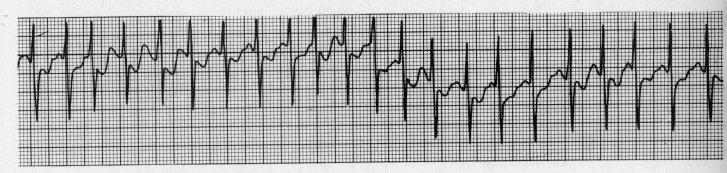

15. Which one of the following is *inappropriate* in treating the above arrhythmia?

   a) Propranolol (Inderal)
   b) Epinephrine
   c) Carotid massage
   d) Digoxin

16. Number the following digitalis preparations in order of rapidity of action and dissipation:

   _____ Digoxin
   _____ Ouabain
   _____ Lanatoside C (Cedilanid)
   _____ Digitoxin

17. Which of the following are contraindications for the use of propranolol (Inderal)?

   a) Heart block
   b) Atrial flutter
   c) Congestive heart failure
   d) Chronic lung disease

18. An elderly patient recovering from a myocardial infarction who is on a maintenance dose of quinidine complains of having "black out" spells. You would suspect:

    a) Postural hypotension
    b) Heart block
    c) Paroxysmal ventricular tachycardia
    d) Small CVAs

19. The nurse's main concern about the digitalized patient who is receiving furosemide (Lasix) is:

    a) Recording I. & O.
    b) Taking CVP readings
    c) Observing for decreasing edema
    d) Observing for arrhythmias due to hypokalemia

20. Cardiac arrest may result from too rapid an infusion of IV phenytoin (Dilantin) because of:

    a) Its depressant effect on the cerebrum
    b) Bradycardia due to the effect of Dilantin
    c) Bradycardia due to the effect of propylene glycol diluent

21. Which of the following drugs, when used in combination with digoxin, increases the serum level of digoxin by 50% to 70%?

    a) Bretylium
    b) Lidocaine
    c) Tocainide
    d) Verapamil

22. Which of the following antiarrhythmic drugs has a half life of 14 to 52 days, making less frequent dosing a possibility?

    a) Amiodarone
    b) Lorcainide
    c) Propafenone
    d) Encainide

Cardiovascular Drugs

ANSWERS TO STUDY QUESTIONS

1. **b** Atropine should be given with a narcotic in the presence of a bradyarrhythmia. Atropine will antagonize the tendency of morphine to increase heart block.
2. **c** This rhythm strip represents atrial fibrillation with an extremely slow ventricular rate and should be regarded as digitalis toxicity. Transvenous pacemaker is the preferred means of stabilizing the patient with severe heart block. In this case, temporary pacing would be needed until the effects of digitalis toxicity disappeared. Potassium chloride will potentiate the toxic action of digitalis when heart block is present, and potassium is contraindicated in this setting. Calcium chloride also aggravates digitalis toxicity.

3. **b** This is a tachyarrhythmia, type unknown, such as can be produced by Isuprel. Lidocaine ordinarily produces no changes in rhythm, and propranolol (Inderal) slows the rate.

4. **d** This is atrial bigeminy with some beats aberrantly conducted. Digoxin is the preferred treatment, but quinidine and propranolol (Inderal) are also effective. Epinephrine will increase irritability.

5. **a** This patient has complete heart block, and IV Pronestyl would be contraindicated, since it could cause ventricular standstill.

6. **d** Perform defibrillation if a defibrillator is immediately available. If not immediately available, a blow to the chest may produce enough electrical discharge to defibrillate the heart (5–10 watt sec). Since this rhythm strip represents ventricular fibrillation, maneuvers such as a, b, or c will only delay proper treatment.

7. **b** This rhythm is atrial fibrillation with a moderately fast ventricular rate. Isuprel will increase the rate further, lidocaine is ordinarily ineffective for this rhythm, and IV quinidine is contraindicated in *any* patient. Digoxin will slow the ventricular rate, may convert the rhythm to a sinus mechanism, and is the drug of choice.

8. **b** Cardioversion. Pacing is ordinarily reserved for abnormally slow rhythms.

9. **d** Yellow vision suggests digitalis intoxication due to a toxic effect of this drug on the retina. A, b, and c are correct for the following reasons:

   1) Fainting may occur from transient ventricular tachycardia or ventricular fibrillation as a *toxic* effect of Pronestyl.
   2) B and c signify development of lupuslike syndrome occurring fairly commonly in patients on Pronestyl.

10. **a** Blood levels are the most accurate means of monitoring the Pronestyl dose since a high level (8 mg/liter) usually correlates with toxicity and a low level (4 mg/liter) is often associated with ineffectiveness in controlling the arrhythmia.

11. **b** Digitalis (and other drugs such as Pronestyl, quinidine, and Inderal) will increase the degree of heart block present.

12. **c** Grand mal seizures are associated with very high levels of lidocaine. Usually an A-V conduction disturbance would also be present.

13. **b** The fourth beat is a ventricular premature contraction (VPC) occurring in a patient with sinus bradycardia. This type of rhythm is commonly seen in the first few hours of infarction. The VPCs usually disappear if the intrinsic heart rate is increased. Atropine will reliably increase the heart rate when sinus bradycardia is present. A pacemaker is usually not necessary unless the rate does not respond to drugs.

14. **c** Propranolol (Inderal). The other drugs increase contractility of the heart.

15. **b** Epinephrine is inappropriate, since it may accelerate the rate further. The rhythm is atrial fibrillation with a rapid ventricular response. Either digoxin or propranolol (Inderal) is likely to be effective. Carotid massage will slow the rate when atrial fibrillation or atrial flutter is present and often will convert paroxysmal atrial tachycardia to sinus rhythm.

16. 1) Ouabain
    2) Cedilanid
    3) Digoxin
    4) Digitoxin

17. **a, c, d** Heart block may be worsened by Inderal, and standstill may result. *C* is a contraindication because Inderal decreases cardiac contractility and will worsen congestive heart failure. Inderal may also be contraindicated in chronic lung disease, since it may accentuate bronchospasm. Atrial flutter often responds favorably to Inderal.

18. **b, c** Both are toxic manifestations of quinidine. Quinidine produces sudden death in 0.5% of patients who use it chronically, and death is due to arrhythmia.

19. **d** Hypokalemia increases the tendency for digitalis toxic rhythms to develop, and potent diuretics such as Lasix and ethacrynic acid, which produce severe potassium loss, should be

used with caution in the patient on digitalis. After a dose of Lasix, 30 to 60 mEq/liter of potassium is lost in the urine.

20. **c** Dilantin should be infused intravenously at a maximum rate of 50 mg/minute.
21. **d**
22. **a**

Percutaneous Transluminal Coronary Angioplasty

STUDY QUESTIONS

1. List three reasons why PTCA can serve as a favorable alternative to coronary artery bypass grafting.

2. State the rationale for giving Persantine and aspirin after PTCA.

3. Explain the rationale for obtaining potassium, creatinine, and blood urea nitrogen (BUN) levels prior to PTCA.

4. List four signs and symptoms of coronary artery occlusion.

5. An intimal dissection which occurs as a result of the dilatation of a coronary artery stenosis will always result in a complication.

                              TRUE   FALSE

6. List three methods of treating angina pectoris.

Percutaneous Transluminal Coronary Angioplasty

ANSWERS TO STUDY QUESTIONS

1. **a)** Risk—or reduced mortality and morbidity
      b) Shorter convalescence with patient's physical capacity following PTCA being as much as 10% greater than those patients undergoing CABG
      c) Lower cost to patient

2. The end result of PTCA upon the intima of a coronary artery may produce slight irregularities potentiating the aggregation of platelets resulting in the formation of a thrombus. Persantine and aspirin contain antiplatelet properties aiding in the prevention of thrombus formation which could result in severe complications.

3. Potassium levels in excess or below normal limits may interfere with the normal electrical conduction system of the heart, resulting in either depressed function or an increased sensitivity and irritability of the myocardium. The changes resulting from hypokalemia or hyperkalemia may be potentiated during PTCA by the temporary ischemia induced while the dilatation balloon is across the lesion and being inflated. The combination of these two variables could give rise to ventricular arrhythmias that may pose a threat to the patient. Elevation in the levels of serum creatinine and/or BUN may indicate problems in kidney function/filtration. It is the kidneys which filter the radiopaque contrast material used to visualize the coronary anatomy during PTCA. One must also be aware of false high levels, particularly BUN, which may only be a reflection of hypovolemia and can be corrected with adequate hydration either intravenously or by mouth.

4. **a)** Angina pectoris
      b) Elevated ST segments and/or T wave inversion

    c) Nausea

    d) Diaphoresis

5. False

6. **a)** Oxygen

    b) Drug therapy

        1) Nitroglycerin po, IV, or IA

        2) Narcotic therapy (Morphine sulfate, Demerol)

    c) Complete bedrest

Intra-Aortic Balloon Counterpulsation

STUDY QUESTIONS

1. Name the four major determinants of myocardial oxygen demand.

2. How does IABP reduce impedance to systolic ejection?

3. How does IABP contribute to decreasing preload?

4. Describe how IABP increases coronary perfusion pressure.

5. What are the contraindications to IABP and why?

6. Why is the assessment of peripheral perfusion of added importance in the patient with an intra-aortic balloon catheter in place?

7. How might late deflation of the balloon be detrimental to cardiac function?

8. Name the five criteria used to assess adequate timing on the arterial waveform.

9. What is wrong with the timing of the balloon on the following waveform?

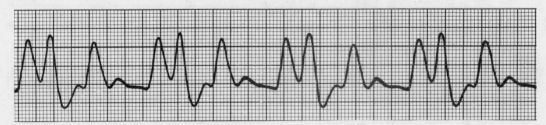

Intra-Aortic Balloon Counterpulsation

ANSWERS TO STUDY QUESTIONS

1. afterload   contractility
   preload   heart rate
2. Deflation of the balloon just prior to systolic ejection displaces a specific amount of volume out of the aorta. Displacement of volume lowers end-diastolic pressure in the aorta, thus decreasing the impedance to ejection.
3. Reduced impedance to ejection improves the forward flow of blood and the ability of the left ventricle to eject its end-diastolic volume. With improved ventricular emptying, there is less back up of blood, so preload is reduced.
4. Inflation of the balloon drives blood flow toward the aortic root in a retrograde manner. Inflation also raises aortic diastolic pressure, thus augmenting the peak pressure during the period of time when coronary artery perfusion takes place.
5. IABP is contraindicated in the following conditions:
   a) *Aortic insufficiency:* The aortic valve must be competent. If aortic regurgitation were present, inflation of the balloon would only serve to increase the amount of regurgitation and exacerbate left ventricular failure.
   b) *Severe peripheral atherosclerotic disease:* This situation interferes with the ability to insert the catheter in the femoral and iliac arteries dut to the occlusive nature of the disease. There is also a danger of damaging vascular tissue that is diseased and possibly ulcerated. The catheter may also possibly disturb a thrombus material that has lodged on the uneven surfaces of the diseased vessels.
   c) *Aortic aneurysm:* Balloon inflation against an aneurysmal sac would promote the dislodgment of aneurysmal debris and precipitate emboli. Insertion of a catheter past an aortic aneurysm would also be dangerous due to the possibility of vascular damage and potential rupture.
   d) *Previous femoral or iliac bypass grafting:* The occluded native vessel would not accommodate the insertion of a catheter. Attempting to pass the catheter through a bypass graft would be relatively impossible due to the required angle of insertion. It might also interfere with the integrity of the graft and would be dangerous due to the possibility of introducing infection.
6. One of the major complications of IABP is vascular insufficiency in the catheterized limb. Perfusion should be frequently assessed for any decrease in circulation to the involved extremity. This should include assessment of skin color, temperature, and peripheral pulses. Capillary refilling following blanching is also an important part of assessing perfusion. In addition, peripheral pulses in the left arm should be noted. Any loss of left arm pulses may indicate obstruction of the left subclavian artery due to improper balloon position.
7. Late deflation of the balloon would elevate end-diastolic pressure in the aorta, possibly beyond what it would be without balloon assistance. This would raise afterload and unnecessarily increase the workload of the heart. Adding increased workload to a ventricle that already is dysfunctional could seriously impair cardiac function.
8. The five criteria are as follows:
   a) Inflation should occur at the dicrotic notch.
   b) The balloon inflation slope should parallel the systolic upstroke.
   c) The diastolic pressure peak should be equal to or greater than the previous systolic peak.

d) An end-diastolic "dip" in pressure should be present.

e) The systolic peak following balloon assistance should be lower than the systolic peak without balloon assistance.

9. Based on the five criteria:

   a) Inflation occurs at the dicrotic notch.

   b) The balloon inflation slope is parallel with the systolic upstroke.

   c) The diastolic pressure peak is greater than the systolic pressure peak.

   d) A diastolic dip in pressure is present, but it does not occur at end diastole. Following the dip, pressure rises and is equal to end-diastolic pressure without balloon assistance. Note the plateau just before the next systolic pressure. This plateau is end-diastolic pressure. In this situation, deflation is too early. The point of deflation should be timed to occur later so that end-diastolic pressure is not allowed to return to normal, unassisted levels. With later deflation, the plateau will disappear.

   e) The systolic pressure peak following balloon assistance is slightly lower than the systolic peak without balloon assistance. With proper balloon deflation, the assisted systolic peak may decrease further.

Autotransfusion

STUDY QUESTIONS

1. CPD (Citrate–Phosphate–Dextrose):
   a) is most commonly used to systemically anticoagulate the surgical patient.
   b) is used routinely to prevent clotting in shed mediastinal blood.
   c) is routinely added to collection reservoirs during emergency and intraoperative ATS procedures.
   d) is a synonym for Heparin.
2. When CPD is indicated, a commonly recommended blood : CPD ratio is:
   a) 7 : 1
   b) 1 : 1
   c) 2 : 1
   d) 20 : 1
3. Defibrinogenated blood:
   a) is collected from the operative site during bypass surgery.
   b) results from contact with serosa or pleural surfaces; for example, shed mediastinal blood.
   c) is always found in conjunction with acute hemothorax.
   d) clotting may be prevented by using the correct CPD ratio.
4. Major hematologic differences between homologous and autologous blood include the following:
   a) Autologous blood has normal levels of 2, 3DPG, a higher platelet count, and a higher hematocrit than homologous blood.
   b) Homologous blood has normal levels of 2, 3DPG, a higher platelet count, and a higher hematocrit than autologous blood.
   c) Autologous blood has normal levels of 2, 3DPG, a lower platelet count, and a higher hematocrit than homologous blood.
   d) Bank blood has normal levels of 2, 3DPG, a higher platelet count, and a lower hematocrit.
5. What is the most frequent complication associated with autotransfusion?
   a) Citrate toxicity
   b) Hemolysis
   c) Microaggregate emboli
   d) Hepatitis

Autotransfusion

ANSWERS TO STUDY QUESTIONS

1. c
2. a
3. b
4. a
5. b

Critical Care Nursing: A Holistic Approach

88

Disseminated Intravascular Coagulation (DIC)

STUDY QUESTIONS

1. DIC is a hypercoagulable syndrome. Explain why patients with this syndrome bleed.

2. Why are platelets reduced in acute DIC?

3. *In vivo*, blood is maintained in a fluid state through the action of coagulation inhibitors. Name the coagulation inhibitors and explain how they inhibit coagulation.

4. Explain how the activation of the fibrinolytic system contributes to the bleeding diathesis in DIC.

5. Explain how heparin controls the progression of coagulation through the intrinsic and extrinsic pathway.

6. Why is the coagulation inhibitor, antithrombin III, unable to regulate the thrombin concentration in DIC?

7. Explain how blood stagnation in the capillary bed favors intravascular clotting.

Disseminated Intravascular Coagulation (DIC)

ANSWERS TO STUDY QUESTIONS

1. DIC is characterized by capillary thrombosis owing to hypercoagulation. The massive capillary network undergoes thrombosis in many organs, consuming clotting factors more rapidly than they can be replenished; hence, bleeding due to clotting factor depletion occurs. Additionally, the activation of the fibrinolytic system results in lysis of clots, producing fibrin degradation products, which further compound the bleeding.
2. Platelets are reduced in acute DIC because they are involved in the capillary thrombotic process and are consumed in the same way that clotting factors are depleted in DIC.

3. a) the liver and the reticuloendothelial system clear activated clotting factors from the blood.
   b) Antithrombin III inactivates thrombin, thus retarding conversion of fibrinogen to fibrin.
   c) Blood flow dilutes activated clotting factors and assists in their removal.
   d) the fibrinolytic system interferes with thrombin at its sites of action on fibrinogen.
4. The lytic enzyme, plasmin, acts to lyze fibrin and fibrinogen and attacks Factor V and Factor VIII, which are required for the activation of Factor X in the coagulation cascade. The lysis of fibrin and fibrinogen results in the liberation of fibrin degradation products (FDP), which interfere with platelet aggregation and have anticoagulant activity.
5. Heparin has an inhibitory effect on the activation of Factor X. Both the intrinsic and extrinsic pathways merge into a final common pathway at activated Factor X. By inhibiting the activation of Factor X, coagulation through either the intrinsic or extrinsic pathway is inhibited.
6. In DIC the excessive thrombin formation that is generated exceeds antithrombin ability to control the thrombin. Also, antithrombin III levels are decreased in DIC.
7. Blood stagnation promotes increased concentrations of activated clotting factors, while the maintenance of an adequate smooth blood flow acts to dilute activated clotting factors and assist in their removal by the liver and reticuloendothelial system.

Respiratory Assessment

STUDY QUESTIONS

1. In what ways does position affect the respiratory functions?

2. What are the clinical manifestations of respiratory failure?

3. List three pulmonary and three nonpulmonary potential causes of respiratory failure.

4. There are several important methods often used simultaneously to monitor adequacy of pulmonary support during continuous mechanical ventilation. One method is arterial blood gas analysis. List three additional methods and briefly state rationale for each.

5. Why are patients who are being suctioned likely to arrest, even though they may have no cardiovascular problems?

6. Define and give the treatment for the following:

    a) Pneumothorax

    b) hemothorax

    c) Tension pneumothorax

7. Why are blood gases important?

8. Mrs. Johnson is a 57-year-old woman who was admitted yesterday with the diagnosis of pneumonia. Today she is being transferred to CCU with the diagnosis of possible ARDS, based on the nurse's evaluation.

    a) What is ARDS and what measures were most likely part of the floor nurse's evaluation?

    b) Upon Mrs. Johnson's arrival in CCU, her physicians are discussing ventilatory support with PEEP. Why?

c) What additional nursing goals will become primary if Mrs. Johnson is placed on a respirator?

Respiratory Assessment

ANSWERS TO STUDY QUESTIONS

1. Standing and semi-Fowler's: Aid respiratory function by increasng the vital capacity primarily because gravity lowers the diaphragm.

   Sitting: The arms weigh approximately 20 pounds and should be supported on chair arms or an overhead table. Saves energy in the work of breathing and allows for chest wall expansion. Permits gravity to move fluids to dependent parts and prevents pooling in pulmonary vascular structures.

   Prone: Abdominal contents move upward, restricting the use of abdominal muscles. Therefore, it is especially poor for emphysematous and other patients who need their abdominal muscles for breathing. The air passages are at a greater right angle, increasing resistance to air flow, and gas distribution is less uniform.

   Side-lying: Restricts chest muscle movement and decreases lung expansion on the side closest to the bed.

2.
Hypoxia	*Hypercarbia*
impaired motor function	headache
impaired judgment	dizziness
confusion, delirium	confusion, delirium
unconsciousness	unconsciousness
decreased tension	asterixis
tachycardia	miosis
central cyanosis	increased tension
vasodilation	tachycardia
(warm extremities)	sweating

3.
Pulmonary causes	*Nonpulmonary causes*
COPD	increased intracranial pressure
asthma	
pneumonia	drug overdose
pneumo/hemothorax	head trauma
flail chest	cervical cord injury
atelectasis	neuromuscular disease
pulmonary emboli	sepsis
ARDS	
abnormalities of bony thorax	

4. Monitor CNS status to elicit the adequacy of oxygenation and ventilation.
   Vital signs will reveal the cardinal signs of hypoxemia and inadequate ventilation.
   Electrocardiographic monitoring detects rhythm disturbances secondary to hypoxemia, inadequate ventilation, and altered acid-base status.
   Pulmonary function studies will evaluate the patient's ability to resume his own ventilatory function.
   Analysis of secretions alerts the nurse to the presence of potential pathogens.

5. Suctioning removes not only secretions, but the patient's oxygen, especially from the "dead spaces." This depletion of O_2 to the brain and heart may cause serious arrhythmias that can lead to ventricular fibrillation. The vagus nerve is also easily stimulated during suctioning. If stimulation of the vagus is severe enough, bradycardia or arrest may occur.

6. a) *Pneumothorax:* Collection of air in the pleural space (the pleural space becomes an actual space)
      Treatment: Depends upon the size of the pneumothorax and may be a simple needle aspiration or a chest tube with underwater seal drainage.
   b) *Hemothorax:* Collection of blood in the pleural space.
      Treatment: A chest tube with underwater seal drainage.
   c) *Tension pneumothorax:* Continual accumulation of air in the pleural space, which does not have the ability to escape (a life-threatening situation).
      Treatment: Immediate aspiration of accumulated air in the pleural space with a 16- or 18-gauge needle, followed by a chest tube and underwater seal drainage.

7. Blood gases are important to determine if the patient is well oxygenated and to determine the acid-base status of the patient.

8. a) ARDS is an acute respiratory distress syndrome believed by many to be caused by alveolar-capillary damage and inability to function. Severe hypoxemia develops with decreased functional residual capacity, intrapulmonary shunting, and decreased lung compliance.

      Measures most likely part of the nurse's evaluation were:
      Vital signs—extremely rapid pulse and respiration
      Sensorium—irritability
      ABGs—increase in PCO_2 and decrease in PO_2
      General appearance of patient
      Notification of physician

   b) To adequately ventilate and oxygenate Mrs. Johnson, PEEP is added. PEEP is positive end expiratory pressure, which is maintained throughout the respiratory cycle. It prevents (or minimizes) alveolar collapse, and gas remains in the alveoli for exchange of O_2 and CO_2 to take place.

   c) Additional nursing goals:
      Monitor ventilatory system for malfunctioning.
      Monitor and maintain patient's respiratory system (airway care and auscultation of chest).
         Prevent complications:
         sterile or clean technique
         nutritional program
         skin and exercise programs
         There are more. What else would you include?

Blood Gases

STUDY QUESTIONS

1. A 25-year-old patient has taken an overdose of drugs and is thought to have vomited and aspirated. The following arterial blood gases were obtained with the patient breathing room air in the Emergency Department:

PO_2	70
PCO_2	60
HCO_3	28

   Using A −a gradients, can you determine if aspiration or other parenchymal lung disease is likely? What caused the hypoxemia?

2. In a postoperative coronary artery bypass graft patient, mixed venous oxygen saturation from a pulmonary artery catheter is 50% and had previously been 65% two hours earlier.

   a) What is the normal range for mixed venous oxygen saturation?

   b) What is the normal range for mixed PO_2?

   c) What are two common causes of falling mixed venous oxygen saturation?

d) What tests should be done to see why mixed venous oxygen saturation is low? Give the rationale for your answers.

Blood Gases

ANSWERS TO STUDY QUESTIONS

1.

PAO_2			minus	PaO_2	=	A − a oxygen gradient
$(760 - 47)\,(.21)$	−	$(1\frac{1}{4})\,(60)$	−	70	=	
$(713)\,(.21)$	−	75	−	70	=	
150	−	75	−	70	=	
75			−	70	=	5

The normal A − a oxygen gradient indicates no parenchymal lung disease and therefore no aspiration. The hypoxemia is caused by hypoventilation, presumably from the drug overdose.

2. **a)** 65%–80%

    b) 35 mm/Hg–49 mm/Hg

    c) **1)** Inability of the lungs to oxygenate arterial blood so that when the tissues extract their normal amount of oxygen, venous blood has a low oxygen content.

        2) Reduction in cardiac output (left ventricular failure) so that tissues must extract an extra amount of oxygen from blood as it slowly traverses tissues leaving the venous blood with low oxygen content.

    d) **1)** *Cardiac output:* to see if it has fallen in comparison to prior cardiac output values.

        2) *Arterial blood gas:* to see if the lungs' ability to oxygenate the blood has deteriorated.

Common Pulmonary Problems

Chronic Obstructive Pulmonary Disease

The patient is a 55-year-old man with emphysema/chronic bronchitis. He is the father of six young children. His wife states that he has been unable to work for the past 2 weeks owing to increasing SOB. In addition, his wife states that his mental alertness has markedly decreased.

History: Patient has had diagnosis of emphysema/chronic bronchitis for 7 years. His work for 30 years has been in a sawmill. He states he has smoked at least 1 package of cigarettes per day for 30 years. He has been on a home pulmonary care program without formal home health care follow-up. He was last seen by a doctor 6 months ago.

Lab values (6 months ago):

Chest x-ray:	unchanged; no infiltrates
ABGs:	pH = 7.35
	pO_2 = 56
	pCO_2 = 60
	HCO_3 = 32

Today's lab values:

Chest x-ray:	cardiomegaly LLL infiltrate
ABGs:	pH = 7.32
	pO_2 = 42
	pCO_2 = 70
	HCO_3 = 18
WBC:	18,000
VS:	B/P 120/80; P 100; RR 32; T 101.8

Admitted to the hospital for evaluation.

STUDY QUESTIONS

1. What is the significance of the laboratory values?

2. What additional information would you like to have?

Doctor's orders include:
>   IPPB with Bronkosol q4h
>   Steam inhalation
>   Postural drainage
>   Vigorous cough
>   Oxygen at 2 L/min

Patient appears to be oriented to surroundings and events.

16 hours later:
>   Patient is very lethargic (in checking O_2 flow-meter you notice flow is at 6 L/min). Breath sounds indicate marked increase in secretions.

3. What action should you take?

24 hours later: Patient is semi-comatose.

>   *ABGs:*
>
> | | | |
> |---|---|---|
> | pH | = | 7.26 |
> | pO_2 | = | 46 |
> | pCO_2 | = | 72 |

Nurses report that the patient is unable to cooperate with bronchial hygiene. Deep nasotracheal suction has been attempted, but was not able to remove a significant amount of secretions. Rhonchi were heard bilaterally in the upper and lower lobes. Respiratory arrest occurred. Patient was intubated, transferred to the ICU, and ventilated for 16 hours. Antibiotic therapy was initiated. Rigorous bronchial hygiene was performed ql–2 hrs. Copious amounts of green-tinged, foul-smelling secretions were suctioned from the endotracheal tube.

Chest x-ray:	decreased infiltrates; cardiomegaly unchanged
ABGs:	oxygen setting at 40%
	pH = 7.35
	pO_2 = 64
	pCO_2 = 48

Patient is oriented and alert.

The endotracheal tube is removed 24 hours later. Rigorous bronchial hygiene is continued. Ambulation is begun.

The patient is transferred from the ICU to the ward 24 hours later.

4. Develop a comprehensive nursing care plan related to patient education for this person.

Chronic Obstructive Pulmonary Disease

ANSWERS TO STUDY QUESTIONS

1. The ABGs reveal hypoxemia and acidemia secondary to alveolar hypoventilation and hypercapnia and metabolic acidosis. Respiratory acidosis existed 6 months ago, but the abnormality has increased. Metabolic alkalosis existed 6 months ago and was probably a compensatory mechanism for respiratory acidosis. At this time the kidneys are not compensating for the respiratory acidosis. The elevated WBC indicates infection. The LLL infiltrate points to infection. Cardiomegaly could be secondary to right heart failure (*cor pulmonale*), caused by the patient's lung disease.

2. **a)** What are the normal ABGs at patient's altitude?
    b) Were first and/or second ABGs drawn when patient was receiving supplemental O_2? If so, how much?
    c) What has home pulmonary care consisted of? How frequently has it been done? Does the patient/family understand the purpose of home pulmonary care? Why wasn't home health care involved?
    d) What patient education has occurred? How much does the patient/family understand about the diagnosis, causative and irritating factors, and therapeutic modalities?
    e) Does the patient know when to call the physician? Does he know where to go for emergency help?
    f) Does the family understand the cardinal signs of respiratory distress? Do they know when to call the physician and where to go in case of emergency?
    g) Are finances a problem? If so, has a social worker been contacted? Is the patient a candidate for Medicaid or Social Security disability?
    h) WBC was 18,000. Would like to have a differential.
    i) Did the patient have cardiomegaly 6 months ago? Chest x-ray report states: "unchanged." (Unchanged from what?)
    j) How significant is shortness of breath (*i.e.,* at rest, performing activities of daily living, or following exercise)?
    k) What medications does the patient take? What is the medication schedule? Does patient/family understand medications, dosage, and side effects?

3. **a)** Decrease O_2 flow to 2 L/min.
    b) Did the patient increase the O_2 flow? Does the patient understand the danger of high-flow O_2? This should be a goal of patient/family education.
    c) Institute rigorous bronchial hygiene therapy, measures to clear secretions. This has been ordered q4h, but has it been rigorous? Need to increase therapy to q2h. Consider suctioning patient if he is not able to cooperate and/or generate an effective cough for secretion clearance.

4. The crucial elements of this nursing care plan should address multiple areas of education, specifying for each the date basic education occurred, how the patient/family demonstrated knowledge, and problem areas. These essential elements are as follows:
    a) Basic airway anatomy
    b) Basic disease process of COPD
    c) COPD may result in:
        1) continuous productive mucus and secretions above normal
        2) decreased natural cleansing mechanism of lungs
        3) decreased size of air passages
        4) increased susceptibility to lung infections

d) Complications of COPD
e) Irritating factors—can make symptoms worse:
   1) smoking
   2) pollution
   3) extremes of weather
   4) household sprays
   5) dust
   6) animal dander
   7) other (specific to patient)
f) Medications—for each:
   1) name
   2) color
   3) description of shape
   4) reason
   5) frequency
   6) dosage
   7) side effects
g) Bronchial hygiene
   1) compressor nebulizer/IPPB
      i) use of
      ii) method of breathing
      iii) method of cleaning
      iv) trouble-shooting equipment
   2) steam inhalation
   3) postural drainage/chest percussion
   4) forceful/effective cough
h) Importance of hydration
   1) contraindications
   2) type of fluids
i) Importance of exercise
j) Exercise program
   1) how much
   2) how often
k) Pursed lip breathing
l) Breathing retraining (if indicated/appropriate)
   1) what
   2) how
m) Indications of pulmonary infection—when to call physician
n) Nutrition
   1) small frequent meals
   2) avoid gas-forming foods
o) Name of your pulmonary doctor
p) Your nurses' names
q) Where to call for any questions or problems related to breathing difficulties
r) Other (specific to patient/family)

Thoracic Trauma

A 65-year-old man was admitted to the emergency room as a result of an auto accident in which he sustained numerous thoracic abrasions and fractured ribs (7 through 11) on the right. The patient was alert and oriented. He was complaining of severe chest pain on inspiration and was very apprehensive.

Vital signs: T 98°F; P 112; R.R. 26; B/P 150/90

Admission Weight: 120 lbs.

Pertinent history: Chronic bronchitis for 15 years which has been treated with intermittent home oxygen, oral bronchodilating agents, steam inhalation, and postural drainage.

STUDY QUESTIONS

1. What information in the above ER report do you consider important? Why?

2. What additional information would you like to have?

The patient was admitted to the hospital. Admission orders included: Demerol 100 mg q4h, prn; Valium 10 mg tid; Nembutal 100 mg hs prn; O₂ prn, and vital signs qid.

The patient continued to be very apprehensive and complained of severe inspiratory chest pain as he was transferred to the ward from the ER.

3. About which of the orders do you have hesitations?

4. Why?

The patient was given Demerol 100 mg and Valium 10 mg at 5 PM and at 9 PM. Vital signs at 11 PM were: B/P 140/90; respirations were shallow at 34/minute; pulse 120/minute. The patient remained apprehensive, but was more comfortable. He asked for oxygen, which he frequently used while sleeping at home. The nurse complied by turning the oxygen on (5 L/min). Nembutal 100 mg was given for sleep.

5. Which of the above actions are inappropriate? Why?

6. What actions would have been more appropriate?

The patient was allowed to sleep until 6 AM. At this time the vital signs were: B/P 164/96; pulse 140/minute; and respirations 54/minute. The patient was confused and diaphoretic.

7. What diagnosis are you considering?

8. What action should you take?

An arterial blood gas sample was drawn on room air at 6:30 AM. The following report was obtained (sea level):

pH = 7.24
pO_2 = 44
pCO_2 = 68
HCO_3 = 24

9. What is your interpretation of these ABGs?

10. What action would you take?

By 10 AM the patient has become combative and uncooperative. Attempts to peform rigorous bronchial hygiene (*i.e.,* inhaled bronchodilator treatments, steam inhalation, postural drainage and chest percussion, forceful coughing and expectoration, and/or suctioning of pulmonary secretions) are futile. ABG results on 70% oxygen delivery system:

pH = 7.22
pO_2 = 40
pCO_2 = 70

11. What action would you take?

12. Why would intubating the patient be considered at this point?

The patient is intubated and placed on a volume respirator. During intubation the patient was noted to have copious green-tinged secretions.

Machine settings (*i.e.,* oxygen, volume, and rate) have been established by the physician. No new orders have been written.

13. How do you assess adequacy of pulmonary support?

14. What are your nursing responsibilities regarding mechanical ventilators (*i.e.,* settings)?

15. What are your priorities for nursing care?

16. What parameters will help you determine that the patient no longer requires ventilatory assistance?

17. Outline the nursing care that will be required after mechanical ventilatory assistance is discontinued.

Thoracic Trauma

ANSWERS TO STUDY QUESTIONS

1. Age is an important consideration. Does the patient have osteoporosis secondary to aging process or steroid therapy? Numerous thoracic abrasions and fractured ribs are an important factor in anticipating pulmonary complications such as pneumothorax, pneumonia, secretion retention secondary to decreased ability to cough forcefully, and atelectasis. Any of these complications could, if severe enough, result in acute respiratory failure. The patient was alert and oriented. Vital signs demonstrated tachypnea and tachycardia—two cardinal signs of hypoxemia; however, these signs can be indicative of other complications. The patient is undoubtedly very thin. Why? Does the patient have poor nutritional status secondary to long-standing chronic lung disease? If so, this will alter the normal healing process and recuperative powers. The past medical history is significant for long-standing COPD requiring supplemental O_2, bronchodilating agents, and measures to clear secretions. The patient presents with a picture of chronic lung disease, which will now be complicated by thoracic trauma that further compromises lung function. This is a potentially disasterous situation. Constant assessment for signs and symptoms indicative of hypoxemia and respiratory failure will be crucial.

2. Was there any other trauma? What are the patient's usual vital signs—at rest and exercise? What is the patient's usual weight? Has there been a significant weight loss? What is the height? How much supplemental O_2 has the patient been receiving? What are the arterial blood gases on room air and with supplemental O_2? What specific bronchodilating agents has the patient been taking? Dosages? How frequently is bronchial hygiene done, and by whom? Is he on any other pharmacologic agents? Does he have a history of chest infections? If so, what is the frequency? Has he ever been in acute respiratory failure? When? Were there any complications (*i.e.,* intubation, ventilatory assistance, cardiac arrest, sepsis, etc.)? Who is the patient's physician? Has he even been hospitalized? If so, where? Does he live with family? Does he have any type of home health care? Any history of heart failure secondary to lung disease? What is history for cough, sputum production, dyspnea, orthopnea, chest pain, smoking, ankle swelling, and hemoptysis?

3 and 4. Demerol, Valium and Nembutal are potential respiratory depressants. The routine administration of any one of these could result in compromised lung function. The combined effects of simultaneous administration could be disasterous and might result in respiratory failure. Question what the specific dosage of supplemental O_2 should be to achieve specific arterial oxygen saturation or arterial oxygen pressure. One should again ask the questions: "What are the patient's usual arterial blood gases? Is he hypoxemic? Does he retain CO_2? What is his bicarbonate level?" The answers to these questions are very important to the nurse who is responsible for monitoring the supplemental O_2 therapy. This is a patient who could quickly develop acute respiratory failure. Tachypnea and tachycardia are cardinal signs of hypoxemia and acute respiratory failure. This knowledge combined with a high index of suspicion for the development of a pulmonary disaster should result in frequent monitoring of vital signs (*i.e.,* hourly for the first few hours. What is the trend?) The final question is whether this patient can be evaluated adequately on the ward. Is there a direct view from the nurses' station plus an adequate staff for provision of care as well as monitoring vital signs, sensorium, etc?

5. A history of chronic lung disease combined with the knowledge that Demerol and Valium are respiratory depressants should alert a nurse to the appropriate administration of these drugs in this patient who weighs only 120 pounds. The fact that the drugs, in significant dosages, were given at 5 PM is a problem. The fact that the same drugs and dosages were repeated 4 hours later should be considered a serious error in judgment. Pre-existing tachycardia and tachypnea have worsened—a bad trend. We do not know what the patient's usual arterial blood gases are. One might assume that a 15-year-history of chronic bronchitis might well be accompanied by chronic hypoxemia and hypercapnia—the latter for unclear reasons. The patient's normal respiratory drive is blunted; therefore, his hypoxic drive is essential. The administration of high-flow O_2 (*i.e.,* 5 L/min) can obliterate the hypoxic drive that is needed for the control of breathing in patients with chronic bronchitis. Nembutal is a potent sedative with respiratory depressant capabilities; it should not have been given.

6. It is important for the nurse to discuss the orders with the physician. The nurse can play an important role in the decision-making process regarding selection of therapeutic modalities for this patient. The patient's long-standing history of chronic bronchitis, which has required bronchodilating agents, supplemental O_2, and measures for secretion clearance should be significant in terms of selecting both pharmacologic agents and dosages, including oxygen. The pain is undoubtedly significant. What is the least amount of pain medication which would minimize the pain? What is the safest agent? What about small doses of Demerol (*i.e.,* 25 mg–50 mg) every 4–6 hours as needed? What about a trial of Talwin or Tylenol for pain control? Before a narcotic is given, be sure to evaluate the vital signs. Does the patient need a sedative for sleep? If so, the safer agent to use, which produces the least respiratory depression, is Dalmané. If Valium is ever used in this type of patient, the dose should be small (*i.e.,* 2.5 mg) and the patient should be monitored carefully for signs and symptoms of respiratory distress.

Oxygen must be ordered in specific concentration or liter flow to accomplish adequate arterial oxygen pressure and/or saturation. Oxygen delivery must then be evaluated at regular intervals.

7. Acute respiratory failure.

8. If RNs are allowed to draw arterial blood gases in an emergent situation without a physician's order, quickly obtain AGBs, send them to the lab, and notify physician of patient's condition. By the time he arrives the ABGs should be ready. In addition, check the oxygen delivery system to ascertain whether it is working properly and whether the delivery device is positioned on the patient correctly. Also, stimulate the patient and assist him in the position which will result in more effective/optimal ventilation. Perform a limited cardiopulmonary exam. What are the breath sounds? Do you hear rhonchi? Bronchial hygiene has been part of the patient's home care program. Have any measures for secretion clearance been initiated during this hospitalization? If not, they should be. There will be some limitations because of the thoracic trauma (*i.e.*, chest percussion over affected ribs). The latter care should be scheduled around the clock. The goal is to improve ventilation and gas exchange. Continue to evaluate the patient carefully for any signs of respiratory failure; note the trend.

9. According to the patient's medical record, the above ABG results represent an acute drop in arterial oxygen pressure accompanied by an acute rise in carbon dioxide pressure with a normal bicarbonate level. Therefore, the diagnosis is acute respiratory failure. The patient has acidemia secondary to alveolar hypoventilation and respiratory acidosis.

10. Continue vigorous bronchial hygiene around the clock and meticulously monitor the vital signs, sensorium, and breath sounds for improvement or further deterioration. Check with the physician for approval to repeat ABGs in 1 hour to document trend. Suggest a partial rebreathing mask for O_2 therapy.

11. Notify the physician that ABGs (give specific results) reveal continued deterioration in spite of rigorous therapy. Be prepared to assist the physician with intubating the patient. Check patient record to be sure that the record reflects the meticulous assessment and care—correlating with appropriate laboratory results—in correct sequence.

12. The degree of hypoxemia is life-threatening; the patient is not responding to current vigorous regime.

13. ABGs in combination with cardiopulmonary assessment.

14. The nurse is responsible for constant monitoring of ventilator to ensure that oxygen concentration, volume, rate, etc. are on appropriate settings. Constant monitoring of the patient is equally essential. Monitor for signs of respiratory distress. Monitor for response to ventilatory assistance.

15. Maintain airway, prevent infection through scrupulous suction techniques and care of the airway; monitor secretions for evidence of infection; continue measures to augment secretion clearance; pay attention to function of each system; know the essential laboratory parameters/trends (*i.e.*, ABGs, CXR, CBC, sputum gram stain and cultures, etc.); know the basic function of ventilator, alarm systems, how to trouble-shoot, and what to do in case of power failure; communicate with patient *and* family.

16. The patient no longer requires ventilatory assistance when ABGs, chest x-ray, minute ventilation, forced vital capacity, negative inspiratory force, and vital signs indicate that pulmonary function is adequate.

17. Until the endotracheal tube is removed, you will need to provide inhaled moisture and suction, to the artificial airway. A regular, around-the-clock schedule for bronchial hygiene should be maintained. Mobilize the patient as quickly as possible and develop a schedule for activities. After the artificial airway has been removed, continue all therapeutic modalities necessary for this patient to optimize/maintain pulmonary function. Patient and family education regarding chronic bronchitis, therapy, and signs and symptoms of complications will be crucial. Both the patient and his family need to understand the importance of regular medical follow-up after hospital discharge. Is home health care needed? Will finances be a concern?

Renal Assessment

STUDY QUESTIONS

1. How would an increase in osmotic pressure in the blood affect the glomerular filtration rate?

2. Describe the mechanism of active transport in the nephron.

3. Describe how sodium concentration is regulated in the kidneys.

4. What is the significance of oliguria?

5. How does decreased cardiac output affect the kidneys?

6. Postural hypotension often occurs in the presence of extracellular volume depletion. Why?

7. How does fluid retention affect CVP?

8. Why may the administration of vasopressors, such as levarterenol (Levophed), reduce renal blood flow?

9. Why does sodium wasting occur during the diuresis stage of renal failure?

10. Why is acidosis likely to occur in renal failure?

11. Why is hyperkalemia likely to occure in the presence of acidemia?

12. What is the mechanism by which ethacrynic acid and furosemide promote the excretion of sodium and potassium?

13. Why is the serum creatinine a more reliable indicator of changes in renal function than the BUN? What additional information does the BUN provide?

14. A patient with congestive heart failure develops oliguria with a low urine sodium concentration. What would you expect his urine osmolarity to be, and why?

15. A 70-year-old woman is admitted with congestive heart failure of recent onset. Her urine output is low (15 ml/hr). The urine sodium is 2.0 mEq/liter and the urine specific gravity is 1.028. The BUN is 36 mg/dl, and the serum creatinine is 1.2 mg/dl. Why is the BUN elevated?

16. A patient in coma with a cerebrovascular accident is found to have a urine output of 5000 ml per day when his intake has been only 2000 ml per day. A plasma osmolality is 320 mOsm/kg and the urine osmolality is 85 mOsm/kg. (BUN and blood glucose are normal.) What is the most likely cause of these findings, and why?

17. A 60-year-old man is admitted to the hospital with a left-sided hemiparesis. He manifests unilateral weakness, but is mentally alert, and his condition appears stable. Forty-eight hours after admission he becomes progressively more obtunded, but there is no change in the degree of his paralysis. Serum chemistries reveal Na, 118 mEq/liter; Cl, 88 mEq/liter; K, 3.6 mEq/liter; CO_2, 20 mEq/liter; and BUN, 4.0 mg/dl. Urine chemistries reveal Na, 22 mEq/liter and osmolality, 320 mOsm/liter. What is the cause of the hyponatremia?

18. What is the mechanism of hyponatremia in patients who are receiving diuretics?

19. Ms. Black, age 50, came in with respiratory distress and a history of Laennec's cirrhosis. During the night, the nurse noticed that Ms. Black's urine output ceased.

    If you were caring for Ms. Black, what other signs, symptoms, and data would you want before making judgments about what to do? What might be happening?

Renal Assessment

ANSWERS TO STUDY QUESTIONS

1. It would decrease the glomerular filtration rate (GFR). The GFR is determined by the fluid and osmotic pressure on both sides of the membrane. An increased osmotic pressure in the blood exerts an increased tendency for the fluid to be held within the blood vessels. Therefore, there would be a lower net filtration pressure, and the GFR would decrease. To illustrate:

   fluid pressure: 70 torr tendency to push fluid out of capillary
                            36 torr tendency to hold fluid in capillary
   osmotic pressure:
                            34 torr total force pushing fluid out

   In addition, the filtrate exerts a fluid pressure against the glomerular membrane, trying to push fluid back into the capillary. In the normally functioning nephron this pressure is 14 torr. Subtracting the 14 torr from the 34 torr gives the net filtration pressure of 20 torr. This is lower than normal, resulting in less fluid being filtered into Bowman's capsule and therefore less urine being excreted.

2. Active transport in the nephron involves the binding of a molecule to a carrier, which then moves the molecule from one side of the membrane to the other. The carrier acts somewhat like a pump, which moves the transported molecule either into or out of a cell. In tubule cells, the carrier is located in the cell membrane nearest the peritubular capillaries, and it transports material out of the tubule cell into the peritubular fluid. This lowers the intracellular concentration of the molecule being transported. This decreased concentration enables more of the molecules to diffuse into the tubule cell. These molecules, in turn, leave the cell and enter the peritubular fluid by means of active transport. This movement of molecules increases the peritubular fluid concentration of the molecule, and this increase, in turn, stimulates the diffusion of the molecule into the peritubular capillaries. Thus, in the nephron, active transport removes molecules from the filtrate (urine) back into the bloodstream.

3. When extracellular fluid concentrations of sodium fall, the adrenal cortex is stimulated to produce aldosterone. The adrenal cortex is stimulated not only by the direct effect of the low sodium, but also by the effect of the kidney, which releases an enzyme called renin. Through a series of conversions to angiotensin II, the adrenal cortex is further stimulated to produce aldosterone, which increases the rate of sodium reabsorption in the distal convoluted tubules.

4. Oliguria, which is defined as a urinary output of 400 ml or less in 24 hours, signifies either functional or anatomic renal impairment. Functional problems, such as hypovolemia, and anatomic causes, such as inflammation, drug toxicity, or tubular necrosis, result in increased water reabsorption and decreased urinary output.

5. Decreased cardiac output results in decreased renal perfusion. When cardiac output falls to the point at which the kidneys' autoregulatory mechanism cannot maintain its own blood flow, the GFR drops, the fluid travels through the tubules more slowly, and water and sodium reabsorption is increased. This is reflected in a decreased urinary output.

6. Postural hypotension is characterized by a marked drop in blood pressure upon standing. Blood pressure is normally maintained during posture changes by pressoreceptors located in arteries such as the arch of the aorta and the internal carotid. These pressoreceptors respond to the amount of pressure within the vessel wall, resulting in adaptation by either vasodilatation or constriction.

   When one changes to a standing position, the size of the intravascular compartment enlarges suddenly because of pooling of blood in the dependent vessels. Normally, the pressoreceptors respond quickly enough to this shift in fluid to maintain blood pressure and prevent fainting.

In extracellular volume depletion there is increased tone in the blood vessels because of decreased volume within the vessels. Therefore the vessels are already at near maximum constriction and are sluggish at responding to further constriction.

7. Fluid overload raises CVP.

8. Levophed causes vasoconstriction, which reduces blood flow throughout the arterial system, including the renal arteries.

9. If the patient has become overhydrated during the shutdown phase of renal failure, a larger amount of fluid will be excreted during the diuretic phase. Because urinary sodium concentration is relatively fixed, the excretion of a large volume of fluid will contain proportionately large amounts of sodium.

10. The kidney is responsible for the excretion of nonvolatile acids, including fixed acids such as phosphates and sulfates. This is probably done through tubular processes, which are impaired in the patient with renal failure.

11. In acidemia there is a higher concentration of hydrogen ion in the body. As a result, the hydrogen ion, which is present in increased amounts in the extracellular fluid, enters the intracellular fluid, exchanging with potassium in order to maintain electrical neutrality. The potassium in turn enters the extracellular fluid causing hyperkalemia.

12. Ethacrynic acid and furosemide block the reabsorption of sodium both in the ascending limb of the loop of Henle and in the distal tubule. In turn there is increased sodium delivery to the site of potassium secretion. This increases the exchange of sodium for potassium and in turn increases potassium losses. If volume depletion occurs with these agents, there is an increase in the release of aldosterone, which further augments the sodium and potassium exchange at this site.

13. The serum creatinine is not as significantly altered by changes in protein intake, catabolic rate, and poor renal perfusion as is the BUN. Changes in serum creatinine concentration, therefore, more accurately reflect true changes in the glomerular filtration rate. The BUN gives additional information in regard to prerenal causes of azotemia and the nutritional status of the individual; a disproportionate increase in the BUN to creatinine ratio suggests increased protein intake, tissue breakdown, or decreased renal perfusion.

14. The individual would have a high urine osmolarity, due mainly to urea, because his kidneys would be avidly reabsorbing sodium and water. The avid sodium and water reabsorption is the result of the kidney's response to the reduced cardiac output and consequent reduced renal blood flow that occurs in this setting.

15. The BUN is elevated disproportionately to the serum creatinine (urea/creatinine = 30/1). In a patient with congestive heart failure this immediately suggests prerenal azotemia due to increased urea reabsorption by the underperfused kidneys.

16. The patient probably has diabetes insipidus, since he is producing large volumes of dilute urine in the face of an increased serum osmolarity. The normal individual would be making large amounts of ADH in an attempt to conserve water with this high a serum osmolarity and would be producing a concentrated urine, which this patient cannot do. Therefore, he is most likely deficient in ADH (diabetes insipidus).

17. This patient manifests the syndrome of inappropriate ADH secretion secondary to cerebrovascular disease. The low BUN suggests volume expansion, and the urinary sodium of 22 mEq/liter and osmolarity of 320 mOsm/liter are higher than one would expect in someone with this degree of hyponatremia. One would expect sodium conservation (<10 mEq/liter) and a very dilute urine. The high sodium in this circumstance is the result of volume expansion, and the high urine osmolarity is due to water retention, both secondary to excess ADH production.

18. Diuretics induce volume depletion by reducing total body sodium. The decreased volume acts as a stimulus to ADH release, overriding the normal osmotic stimuli. Decreased blood volume also results in increased proximal tubular sodium and water reabsorption, and the excess ADH results in water reabsorption distally, causing hyponatremia. This sequence of events is more likely to occur in someone who already has a decreased effective blood volume, as in conges-

tive heart failure or cirrhosis, and who receives diuretics without simultaneous water re- striction.

19. Compare the amount of intake to the output, considering such sources of loss as fever; gastrointestinal losses; increased activity; hot, dry environment; hyperventilation; and perspiration. Observe the trend of output, the urine concentration, osmolarity, specific gravity, and odor. Look for signs of thirst, skin turgor, dryness, firmness, and dependent edema. Listen to chest sounds for indications of congestion. Check blood pressure—trend; pulse—rate and quality; heart—apical rate, third or fourth sound. Check CVP or jugular vein distention. Check administration of drugs affecting either conservation or loss of fluid, such as steroids, diuretics. Without the above information, it is difficult to know the cause of Ms. Black's anuria. She may be dehydrated because of inadequate fluid intake, and thus her kidneys are conserving fluid, or she may be experiencing fluid retention from congestive heart failure and inadequate renal perfusion. By knowing the above data, however, one can take appropriate action. In actuality, Ms. Black had symptoms of dehydration with a CVP of 0.

Dialysis

STUDY QUESTIONS

1. Explain the principle by which metabolic waste products are removed in dialysis.

2. What prevents blood cells from crossing the dialyzing membrane?

3. What is the etiology of acidosis in the uremic patient? How is acidosis corrected both before and during dialysis?

4. How does protein intake differ between the nondialyzed uremic patient and the patient who is on a dialysis regimen?

5. List four situations that can contribute to hyperkalemia in the patient with acute renal failure.

6. Why are femoral catheters a first choice over arteriovenous (AV) shunts and fistulas for an acute dialysis?

7. Why do femoral catheters require more careful observations by the nurse during dialysis than either the AV shunt or fistula?

8. Why should a person who has an AV shunt carry shunt clamps at all times?

9. Why does a shunt infection present a potentially serious problem for the dialysis patient?

10. How can the nurse evaluate the cause of shunt clotting?

11. How can the nurse determine whether the artery or the vein is responsible for a deteriorating blood flow rate during and after hemodialysis?

12. If shunt failure occurs during dialysis, how can the procedure be continued?

13. Why is it essential to keep dialysate sterile in peritoneal dialysis and not in hemodialysis?

14. Why is it better to control hypertension with sodium and fluid restriction rather than with drugs?

15. Why does hypotension during hemodialysis sometimes occur in a patient who has fluid overload?

16. How does the nurse decide how much fluid a patient should lose during hemodialysis?

17. Why is weight a more accurate guide than blood pressure for assessing ultrafiltration during hemodialysis?

18. During hemodialysis, what symptoms suggest disequilibrium syndrome?

19. Are intravenous fluids given routinely to combat hypotension?

20. How would the nurse go about assessing the causes of nausea and vomiting during dialysis?

21. What steps does the nurse take in a blood-leak alarm?

22. How does the nurse go about evaluating the cause of chills and fever during hemodialysis?

23. Incomplete recovery of fluid is a technical complication of peritoneal dialysis. What signs and symptoms will alert the nurse to this problem?

24. Peritonitis is a serious but manageable complication of peritoneal dialysis. List three symptoms of perionitis.

Dialysis

ANSWERS TO STUDY QUESTIONS

1. Dialysis is based on the principle of diffusion, which is the tendency of dissolved ions and molecules to distribute themselves evenly throughout a solution. If a membrane is placed between two fluid compartments (blood and dialysate), the particles small enough to pass through the membrane will move from an area of high concentration to one of lower concentration. For example, during dialysis, urea, which is in high concentration in the blood compartment, will move with the dialysate, which contains no urea.

2. The pore size of the membrane permits particles of low molecular weight to pass through the dialyzing membrane easily. Waste products, such as urea and creatinine, which cross the dialyzing membrane, have molecular weights in the hundreds, while protein molecules, which include red blood cells and bacteria, have molecular weights above 50,000 and will not pass through the membrane.

3. Acidosis occurs in the uremic patient because the kidneys cannot excrete the acids formed during normal body metabolism. The body uses bicarbonate to buffer the acids, but as uremia progresses, the supply is depleted and must be replenished. In the predialysis stage, sodium bicarbonate is administered either orally or intravenously. During hemodialysis, either bicarbonate or acetate is added to the bath. Acetate diffuses into the blood where it is converted to bicarbonate.

4. Protein is restricted in the uremic patient to minimize urea production and to prevent excessive accumulation in the bloodstream. This is done in spite of the fact that a restricted protein intake leads to progressive tissue wasting and weight loss. However, once dialysis is initiated, the protein intake is increased to normal levels, since regular hemodialysis treatments will keep blood urea levels in an acceptable range.

5. Any massive tissue destruction, such as burns and crushing injuries, that results in the release of potassium from the damaged cells into the bloodstream can cause hyperkalemia in renal failure. Blood transfusions resulting in hemolysis and potassium-containing drugs can also cause hyperkalemia in the patient who is unable to excrete the excessive potassium.

6. Femoral catheters are usually employed for an acute dialysis where time is an important factor. Both an AV shunt and an AV fistula require the services of a skilled surgeon as well as operating room facilities. It is advisable not to use these systems immediately because of the possibility of bleeding and spasm. In addition, the AV fistula often necessitates waiting several days and even weeks before the vessels become sufficiently dilated.

7. Because of their placement in the groin, the femoral catheters are not readily visualized by the nurse or the patient. Since the patient may be acutely ill and restless, accidental dislodging is more of a risk.

8. If the cannulas accidentally separate, serious blood loss will occur unless they are immediately clamped. The cannulas should then be reconnected and unclamped. If the arterial cannula slips out of the vessel, apply direct pressure until medical assistance is available.

9. Because a shunt is placed directly into the blood stream and is handled and manipulated many times in the normal dialysis routine, it is subject to infection. Once the shunt becomes infected, the risk of septicemia is great. Antibiotic therapy poses a further problem, since many drugs cannot be given because they are excreted through the kidneys. In addition, repeated shunt infections may require surgical revisions, and the patient can conceivably run out of adequate blood vessels.

10. Observe the shunt for signs of infection, since the induration and subsequent pressure on and constriction of the vessel can lead to clotting. Check for shunt alignment, since misalignment hinders blood flow. Assess the patient's recent blood pressure readings to ascertain whether or not hypotension and the concurrent reduced blood flow are causing the clotting. Question the patient about his activities. For example, did he bump or in some way injure the shunt site? Did he sleep with his arm flexed? Both situations can cause reduced blood flow. Since chilling can lead to constriction of blood vessels and slowing of blood flow through the shunt, ask whether or not he has been out in cold weather.

11. Observing the pressure in the drip chamber will help determine which vessel is causing the problem. If the vein is obstructed by a clot or a mechanical defect, there will be increasing resistance to the returning blood, which will trigger the high pressure alarm. In addition, the patient may feel pressure and pain in the vessel. On the other hand, insufficient flow from the artery will result in a low pressure alarm. The arterial blood line will collapse and feel soft, and air will be drawn into the blood line.

    If a shunt clots after dialysis, the ease with which each cannula is declotted will tell the nurse which of the vessels is causing the problem. When the flow from the artery is less than brisk, the artery is probably at fault. On the other hand, when the vein cannot be irrigated easily and the nurse feels resistance in the vessel, the vein is obstructed.

12. If the artery is the cause of the shunt failure and dialysis cannot be postponed, the femoral artery can be catheterized and used as a blood source. The blood can be returned through the venous cannula. If the problem is in the vein, the nurse can do a venipuncture in any vein large enough to take the 14-gauge fistula needle and return the blood in that manner. The venous cannula should be irrigated with heparinized saline during the procedure to preseve the vessel for possible shunt revision.

13. The peritoneal dialysate comes in direct contact with the peritoneum, which is vulnerable to infection. However, in hemodialysis, the cellophane membrane separates the dialysate from the patient's blood, and bacteria are too large to cross the cellophane membrane.

14. The use of antihypertensive drugs can complicate the course of the dialysis by producing hypotension during the treatment. This is especially true when the drug is given just before the dialysis is started. Hypotension interferes with the process of ultrafiltration and therefore with the removal of fluid during dialysis. On the other hand, adequate sodium and fluid restriction

will control hypertension in most patients and not only will permit a smoother dialysis, but also will avoid the complication of fluid overload.

15. Fluid is removed from the vascular compartment during hemodialysis. Because it takes time for the interstitial fluid to move into the circulating fluid, the patient may become hypovolemic as a result of rapid and excessive ultrafiltration. To avoid hypotension, excess fluid should be removed gradually.

16. In making her decision, the nurse uses such data as dry weight, weight gain since the last dialysis, blood pressure, and presence or absence of symptoms of fluid imbalance. For example, a patient comes in for dialysis weighing 70 kg. His weight at the end of his last dialysis 2 days ago was 68 kg, which is also his dry weight. Today his blood pressure is at the upper range of normal for him. The nurse decides that the patient is 2 kg over his dry weight. At this point, because response to fluid removal varies among patients, a knowledge of the patient's usual dialysis course will assist the nurse in deciding whether to remove the entire 2 kg in one dialysis or to spread the removal over several dialyses.

If the patient has not tolerated excessive fluid removal in the past or does not seem to be tolerating it during the current dialysis, the nurse may decide to remove only 1.5 kg at present, caution the patient not to gain over 0.5 kg until the next dialysis, and remove the remaining 0.5 kg at the next dialysis. On the other hand, if the patient has some suggestion of fluid overload such as edema or shortness of breath, it is mandatory to remove at least 2 kg and perhaps 3 kg.

17. Weight is an accurate reflection of how much fluid the patient is losing, whereas blood pressure may reflect and be influenced by other factors. For example, the patient may have been given a sedative or tranquilizer, which may cause a drop in blood pressure.

18. Nausea, vomiting, headache, restlessness, and hypertension are often mild symptoms of disequilibrium. Exacerbation of the mild symptoms plus severe restlessness, twitching, and convulsions indicates severe disequilibrium.

19. No. Sometimes lowering the head of the bed and reducing the blood flow rate and ultrafiltration rate will restore the blood pressure to normal.

20. There are many reasons that patients have nausea and vomiting during dialysis. For example, they are sometimes an early sign of hypotension, while in the presence of hypertension they may be the result of disequilibrium. Anxiety, especially in a new patient, can result in vomiting after meals, indicating the need to feed patients lightly for the first few dialyses. Nausea and vomiting following medication may indicate drug intolerance.

In determining cause and effect as a prerequisite for nursing intervention, it is necessary to find out as much about the symptoms as possible. Useful data include determining when the symptoms began, how many episodes the patient has had and whether or not they are getting better, what they are like and how severe, and at what time of day and in relation to what activity or situation they occur. This information will serve as a basis along with other objective data upon which to make a nursing judgment.

21. First she should check the dialysate with a hemastix to make sure it isn't a false alarm. If gross blood is not visible but the hemastix is positive, the nurse may decide to watch the leak for 15 or 20 minutes, since minor leaks sometimes seal over. However, a minor leak may progress rapidly to a major leak, resulting in a large blood loss. Therefore, if the leak persists beyond 15 to 20 minutes, it is safer to discontinue the dialysis and restart it with another dialyzer.

22. Mild chilling and mild fever can be the result of extremes in the dialysate temperature, so the bath temperature should be checked first. It is not uncommon for a patient to have a temperature of 99° or 99.4°F (37.2° or 37.4°C) if the dialysate temperature reaches 100°F (37.8°C). However, chills and fever could also be the result of septicemia secondary to another infection, or of pyrogenic contamination of dialysis equipment. An obvious source of infection such as the shunt might be present. In any case, blood cultures should be drawn routinely. In the absence of an infection, an examination of the extracorporeal circuit should be made. Inflow and outflow dialysate and dialysate supply tanks should be cultured. Bacteria in the dialysate are too large to cross the membrane, but if the bacterial count is high (over one million per

ml), bacterial toxins can diffuse into the blood. Contamination of a central delivery system is confirmed if more than one patient becomes symptomatic in the same day. Pyrogenic reactions are usually of short duration and respond to the administration of antihistamines and antipyretics.

23. Abdominal distention, complaints of fullness, a difference of 500 ml or more between the amount of fluid inserted and the amount returned (*i.e.,* drainage returned is 500 ml less than amount inserted), hypertension, and other symptoms of fluid overload may occur. Weight is an accurate reflection of the amount of fluid unrecovered.

24. Low-grade fever, abdominal pain when fluid is being inserted, and cloudy peritoneal drainage fluid are symptoms of peritonitis.

Renal Transplantation

STUDY QUESTIONS

1. Ms. James is 6 months post-transplant. In a routine outpatient visit, a bruit, not previously present, is heard lateral to the midline and medial to her kidney. She is taking propranolol, 20 mg qid, and has had well-controlled blood pressures (116–124/80). Today her BP is 150/94, and her serum creatinine has risen from 1.1 mg/dl to 1.9 mg/dl. What might you consider as the etiology of these changes and why?

2. A patient who received a cadaver kidney transplant was oliguric after surgery and did not begin producing urine until the seventh postoperative day. What is the most probably cause of this delay in urine output?

3. Mr. Johnson is 10 days post-transplant. His daily urine output has been 2400 to 3000 ml since his transplant, with 8-hour outputs of 800 to 1000 ml. During his tenth postoperative night his total output is 150 ml. What are the possible causes for this drop in output? What information would you gather and why?

4. A patient who yesterday received a transplant from a living related donor is now having intermittent gross hematuria. A Foley catheter is in place, and hourly urine outputs have ranged from 125 to 200 ml. Suddenly, the hourly urine output decreases to 20 ml. Is this to be expected? Why or why not?

5. Why is a renal transplant generally more successful with a living related donor graft than with a cadaver donor graft?

6. In any phase of transplant patient care, which extremity should be used for blood pressure readings, venipunctures for blood drawing, and starting intravenous fluids? Why?

7. Why is it important for the nurse caring for a new postoperative transplant patient to know whether or not the patient's own kidneys are present and, if so, how much urine they produce daily?

8. Ms. L. received a 2-antigen matched cadaver kidney. Ms. L. still has her native kidneys in place. Since the operation, she has had a small but consistent urine output of 10 to 20 ml every hour. For which electrolyte imbalance should the nurse be especially alert? Why?

9. Peter received a renal graft from his father. Initially he had problems with bladder spasms and hypertension (180/100). Although output is good (2400 ml/day), Peter has had a long history of hypertension, and after transplant he is placed on antihypertensive drugs (hydralazine [Apresoline] and methyldopa [Aldomet]) in increasing doses. On the second postoperative day his BP is 120/100. Are you concerned about his change in blood pressure? If so, what other information will you collect?

10. For each characteristics of rejection, categorize according to the classification of rejection.
    Classifications of Rejection
    1) Accelerated
    2) Acute
    3) Chronic
    4) Hyperacute
    Characteristics of Rejection
    _____ **a)** does not always require nephrectomy
    _____ **b)** may take a year or longer
    _____ **c)** most common form
    _____ **d)** occurs after first week posttransplant
    _____ **e)** occurs during first week posttransplant
    _____ **f)** occurs less than 1% of the time
    _____ **g)** occurs within 24 hours of the transplant
    _____ **h)** reversible with treatment
    _____ **i)** second most infrequent type of rejection

11. For each medication effect, identify the medicine(s) which cause(s) it.
    Medicine
    1) Prednisone
    2) Imuran
    3) Cytoxan
    4) ATB/ALG
    5) Cyclosporine
    Medication Effects
    _____ **a)** anaphylaxis
    _____ **b)** Cushing's syndrome
    _____ **c)** diabetogenic
    _____ **d)** fever
    _____ **e)** hair loss
    _____ **f)** hemorrhagic cystitis
    _____ **g)** hepatotoxic
    _____ **h)** hirsutism
    _____ **i)** leukopenia
    _____ **j)** local reaction or phlebitis
    _____ **k)** nausea/vomiting/bloating
    _____ **l)** nephrotoxic
    _____ **m)** tremors
    _____ **n)** ulcerogenic

Renal Transplantation

ANSWERS TO STUDY QUESTIONS

1. An elevated serum creatinine and blood pressure may well be indicative of a rejection episode or of toxicity from cyclosporine. However, the distinguishing feature of Ms. James' symptoms is the appearance of an abdominal bruit, suggestive of renal artery stenosis. The development of the bruit is a function of the swishing of blood through the narrowed lumen of the artery. This decreased perfusion to the kidney leads to increased renin production, causing further elevation of the blood pressure. Renal function may deteriorate as a result of decreased perfusion as well.

2. Acute tubular necrosis is the result of ischemic injury to the kidney. If the donor nephrectomies are done on a patient who has died from a cardiac arrest, the period of ischemic injury is longer than it is in nephrectomies done on a patient pronounced dead on the basis of brain death and whose cardiovascular function is being maintained. In either situation, there is some inevitable ischemic injury to the organ between the time of procurement and transplantation, which causes tubular injury and may result in delayed recovery of function.

3. The possible causes of Mr. Johnson's drop in output are:

   a) Hypovolemia
   b) Acute rejection episode
   c) Technical complications

   The nurse should first check the previous day's intake and output record to make sure Mr. Johnson is not dehydrated. In addition, the nurse should recheck urine specific gravity, blood pressure, and skin turgor to aid her assessment of the hypovolemic status. If Mr. Johnson is well hydrated, the next assessment should ascertain the possible presence of an obstruction of urinary flow. This may include a sonogram to rule out any technical or mechanical obstructions and assure that the bladder is emptying properly. Once this has been satisfied, the nurse should observe for symptoms that may indicate the beginning of an acute rejection episode, which frequently starts from the seventh to the twenty-first day posttransplant.

   To assist her assessment of rejection episode, the nurse should gather the following information:
   a) Previous day's weight (A weight gain of more than 2 pounds a day is unacceptable and indicates either fluid overload or decreased graft function.)
   b) Peripheral, sacral, or incisional edema (If only incisional edema is present, a pelvic lymphocele should be considered.)
   c) Fever (100°F or 37.8°C or more)
   d) Increased blood pressure
   e) General malaise, irritability
   f) Increase in the size of the transplanted kidney
   g) Tenderness over the transplant
   h) Increased serum creatinine and urea nitrogen
   i) Decreased urine creatinine
   j) Decreased creatinine clearance
   k) Possible decreased urine sodium

4. A drop in urine output is not expected on the first postoperative day unless the intravenous fluids have not been running at the prescribed rate and the patient has become dehydrated. The nurse should then check the Foley catheter and tubing to make sure they are not kinked

and that their position is not interfering with drainage. The likely cause of decreased output is a clot associated with the hematuria, partially occluding the lumen of the Foley catheter. If the patient is well hydrated and the catheter is patent, next check the abdominal dressings to see if the amount of drainage has suddenly increased. Supersaturated abdominal dressings may indicate a ureteral leak, an early technical complication of transplant surgery. A decrease in output associated with rejection is not expected until the seventh to tenth postoperative day unless it is hyperacute/accelerated rejection.

5. A graft from a living related donor is *generally* more successful because the chances of obtaining a good tissue match are greatest within the immediate family structure. This schematic drawing shows the basic concepts of possible tissue antigens within the family structure. This is a simple model and does not represent actual antigens or the complete MHC compatibility complex. Each number represents an antigen, and each vertical pair of numbers symbolizes a haplotype.

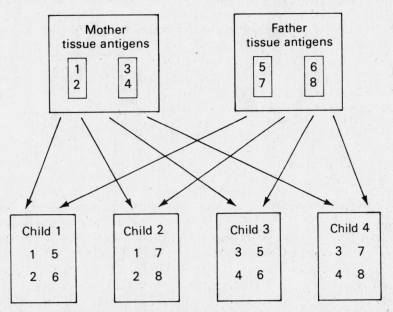

The diagram shows that a parent-to-child graft always provides a 1-haplotype match, since the child inherits one set of tissue antigens from each parent. A sibling graft has the potential (25% chance) of providing an identical match with both haplotypes the same. It also has a 25% chance of providing a total mismatch, in which no tissue antigens are the same, and a 50% chance of a 1-haplotype match. An identically matched graft is the optimal choice for graft survival, but even this best match does not guarantee success, since a small percentage (5%) of these transplant grafts are rejected for as yet unknown immunologic reasons. In addition to the tissue antigen compatibility, ABO compatibility is also necessary.

6. The extremity that should be used for blood pressures, venipunctures, or stafling IVs in any transplant patient is the one without a functioning vascular access site. Even momentary occlusion of blood flow may initiate the clotting mechanism and either decrease the rate of flow or occlude the access site. A functioning access site is necessary in case a rejection episode requires dialysis.

7. Knowing whether or not the patient has his own kidneys and, if so, their approximate output, helps the nurse judge after transplant how much the transplanted kidney is contributing to urinary output.

8. The nurse should observe for hyperkalemia because, regardless of the fluid output of Ms. L's own kidneys, there will be poor solute clearance with her minimal urine output. The surgical trauma causes release of potassium from the intracellular space to the intravascular volume,

which cannot be adequately removed from the blood due to poor renal filtration. Hyperkalemia is a life threatening complication and requires immediate intervention.

9. Since Peter has a long-standing history of hypertension and has remained hypertensive in spite of therapy, a sudden drop in the systolic pressure should arouse some curiosity and concern. The nurse should examine the patient, particularly his transplant wound, for any evidence of bleeding. A fullness in the wound is indeed a finding that should be reported, since Peter may slowly be losing blood from a small bleeding vessel, which would be collecting around the kidney. Even if the findings are unremarkable, the physician should be informed of the blood pressure change, since there remains the possibility that blood could be collecting posterior to the kidney in a way that it cannot be detected until far more blood collects in the perinephric area.

This drop in blood pressure is not a function of antihypertensive medications but is due to a loss of volume. Therefore, the nurse should check for other signs of hypovolemic shock, such as increased pulse and respiratory rate.

10.
   a) 3
   b) 3
   c) 2
   d) 2
   e) 1
   f) 4
   g) 4
   h) 2
   i) 1

11.
   a) 4
   b) 1
   c) 1, 5
   d) 4
   e) 2, 3
   f) 3
   g) 2, 5
   h) 5
   i) 2, 3, 4
   j) 4
   k) 5
   l) 5
   m) 5
   n) 1

Neurologic Assessment

STUDY QUESTIONS

1. Is the plasma hypertonic in association with hyponatremia in the SIADH secretion? Explain.

2. Does administration of sodium chloride-rich intravenous fluids benefit an individual with SIADH? Explain.

3. What would you observe and record in a patient admitted from a car accident with possible head injury?

4. What would you do if you noticed a change in respirations in a patient with a possible head injury? Why?

5. How can fatigue affect the response to testing for level of consciousness?

6. What is wrong with this nursing observation: "Patient responds to stimuli with movement"?

7. Following a grand mal seizure you note the patient's grasp in his right hand to be much weaker than that of his left hand, a condition that was not present prior to the onset of the seizure. The patient is also unable to lift his legs off the bed but is able to move them to some degree. What condition might explain these findings? What action should you take?

8. List the signs and symptoms that indicate a rise in intracranial pressure.

9. In completing a cranial nerve check on an 18-year-old auto accident victim, you note that his tongue has a slight tremor and also deviates to the right. What might this indicate? What action, if any, would you take?

10. You are caring for a patient with a left CVA. Draw the visual pathways involved and explain why and where you would look for hemianopsia. Would you expect this patient, who was left-handed before his illness, to have aphasia or agnosia?

11. You are caring for a patient with bitemporal hemianopsia not caused by glaucoma. Show were there is interference with the visual pathways and speculate on the most common cause for this problem. What would be an appropriate nursing action? How do you envision this disability affecting the patient?

12. A head-injured patient has the following neurologic dysfunctions. What symptoms would you expect to find, and what nursing measures would you institute?
    a) Pyramidal tract damage as shown by a positive Babinski's reflex on the right
    b) Lack of sensation by the right upper extremity
    c) Facial nerve damage on the left
    d) Trigeminal nerve damage on the left
    e) Hypoglassal nerve dysfunction on the left

Neurologic Assessment

ANSWERS TO STUDY QUESTIONS

1. No. The plasma is hypotonic while the urine is hypertonic. The hypotonicity of plasma is representative of water retention.
2. Only transiently, if at all. Treatment consists most importantly of fluid restriction.
3. Level of consciousness
   Motor function and sensation of all extremities
   Size and reaction of pupils

Vital signs—blood pressure, pulse, respirations, temperature
Orientation
Airway and ventilation status
Urinary output
Any indications of CSF leak
Functional status of the 12 cranial nerves

4. A change in the respiratory pattern of a patient with a possible head injury may indicate pathology in the respiratory center in the medulla. This is a serious development and, if possible, medical measures must be instituted to stem its progression, including measures to reduce cerebral edema and to rule out hematoma. Blood gases would be helpful in determining the presence of acidosis or alkalosis, both of which may cause secondary brain damage. Nursing action to secure an adequate airway, such as positioning and removing secretions, is imperative.

5. Fatigue may result in the patient's sluggish response to sensory and verbal stimuli. However, with adequate stimulation the fatigued patient *can be aroused* in order to evaluate his neurologic status. It is imperative that the nurse distinguish between the patient whose response is sluggish because of fatigue and the patient whose response is diminished as a result of intracranial pathology.

6. It does not provide sufficient data for comparing subsequent evaluations. Specific information regarding the type and degree of stimulation used and the specific response elicited must be recorded.

7. The condition is most likely Todd's palsy, the temporary paralysis or paresis that sometimes occurs following a grand mal seizure. Reassure the patient and continue to observe for any change, notifying the physician if the situation does not improve.

8. Any change in the level of consciousness would be the first indication of a rise in intracranial pressure. (Increasing alertness should not be interpreted as improvement until other factors can support this, such as stable vital signs, equal and reactive pupils.) Systolic blood pressure elevation accompanied by widening pulse pressure and slow bounding pulse is a classic sign. Pupillary changes, such as ipsilateral dilatation or bilateral fixation and dilatation, are also important signs.

9. Tremor and deviation of the tongue indicate damage to the hypoglossal nerve, XII, and point to the presence of a lesion on the right side of the brain. The physician should be notified at once, and neurological checks done every 10 to 15 minutes.

10.

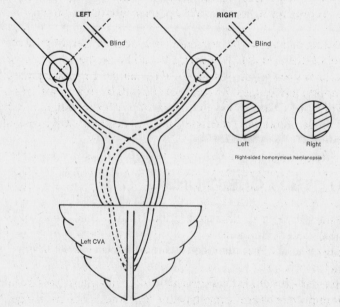

The patient with a left CVA (motor deficit on the right, if present) is shown by the opposite diagram. Because this patient was left-handed, his dominant cerebral hemisphere should have been on the right and unaffected. (However, left-handed people are not as likely as right-handed people to have the dominant hemisphere on the opposite side of the brain.) If this individual followed the usual physiological pattern, he would be more likely to have some form of agnosia than aphasia.

11.

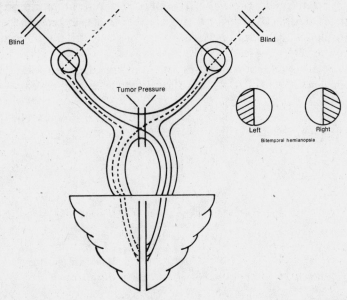

The most common neurologic cause for bitemporal hemianopsia (shotgun, barrel, or tunnel vision) is a pituitary tumor that exerts pressure on the optic chiasm. The patient needs to know about his decreased peripheral vision laterally. He can be taught to turn his head and scan his visual fields. When looking for objects, he simply must broaden his field of search. His visual deficit would not likely be combined with agnosia, and therefore should not be as much of a problem as the hemianopsia that afflicts the stroke patient.

If his visual deficit is permanent and severe, this patient may not be able to drive safely. Lack of peripheral vision may hinder one in his occupation, although it often can be compensated for nicely. The accompanying problems of a pituitary tumor will be more troublesome than the visual deficit.

12. a) Pyramidal tract damage yields voluntary motor deficit. Because the pyramidal tracts cross at the level of the medulla, the damage would be on the left side of the brain. This is an upper motor neuron lesion, which would usually yield a spastic paralysis making exercise doubly important. Weakness or paralysis needs to be treated with proper body alignment and support, preventing stress or subluxation of joints. Alignment in conjunction with complete range of motion exercises as often as necessary will maintain a flexible limb for rehabilitation.

b) Lack of sensation in conjunction with cerebral damage indicates brain damage on the opposite side of deficit. Sensory loss should be evaluated in relation to the rest of the patient's neurologic status and any evidence of decrease or increase. Loss of sensation makes the joints susceptible to stress, and poor alignment or support may go unnoticed. Certainly the loss of defensive mechanism must be considered in protecting the patient from burns, pressure, and so forth. One should also observe for evidence of missed trauma due to lack of pain (fractures or lacerations especially). Finally, in rehabilitating the patient, lack of sensation calls for teaching measures regarding protection of the extremity.

c) Facial nerve damage would be indicated by loss of the muscles of facial expression. Noting the loss is important to evaluating baseline function, as well as change. The ability to blink with the upper eyelid may or may not be affected. Eye care to prevent drying and scarring of the cornea is indicated when blinking ability is lost or decreased. The patient may need assistance in eating or in dietary change due to drooping of the mouth.

d) Trigeminal nerve damage causes loss of the muscles of mastication, sensory loss to the face, and can yield loss of corneal reflex. Loss of the muscles of mastication would affect chewing. Sensory loss requires consciousness of the loss of defense both by the nurse and the patient for maximum protection. Loss of corneal reflex requires protection of the eye when danger of foreign bodies or drying of the cornea is increased. The appropriate plan for protecting the eye would need to be worked out with the physician, and the nurse would then teach the patient.

e) Hypoglossal nerve dysfunction causes loss of motor function of the tongue. This would hinder chewing and increase the need for mouth care on the weak side.

Invasive Neurologic Assessment Techniques

STUDY QUESTIONS

1. Cerebral Perfusion Pressure (CPP)

   a) often increases with suctioning.
   b) provides a clinical estimate of cerebral blood flow.
   c) has a normal range of 11–15 mm Hg.
   d) is the difference between the systolic and diastolic ICP.

2. Initial treatment for increased intracranial pressure usually includes which of the following?

   a) Craniectomy
   b) Induced barbiturate coma
   c) Pancuronium or curare
   d) Diuretics, steroids, hyperventilation, and CSF drainage

3. Clinical signs and symptoms of supratentorial herniation

   a) provide an early warning of impending increases in intracranial pressure.
   b) are usually reversible.
   c) if present, are usually preterminal.
   d) usually occur after the intracranial pressure has exceeded 25 mm Hg.

4. Normal intracranial pressure is

   a) 50 to 60 mm Hg.
   b) 11 to 15 mm Hg or less.
   c) 20 to 40 cm of water.
   d) approximately the same as mean systemic arterial blood pressure.

5. Induced barbiturate coma

   a) should be preceded by ICP, BP, PA, EGG monitoring, baseline recordings, and assisted ventilation.
   b) produces the same clinical results as the use of pancuronium.
   c) is usually initiated shortly after the patient's ICP exceeds 15 mm Hg.
   d) contraindicates the use of hypothermia.

6. Nursing measures which may prevent or reduce IICP include which of the following?

   a) Frequent suctioning with aggressive hyperventilation
   b) Flushing ICP line q1h and PRN
   c) Elimination of extracranial causes of IICP
   d) Frequent turning and repositioning

7. Most adult ICUs currently doing ICP monitoring use which of the following?

   a) Intraventricular catheters
   b) Subarachnoid screws
   c) Epidural devices
   d) A combination of intraventricular and subarachnoid methods

8. Continuous flush devices are not used for ICP monitoring because

   a) a small increase in the volume of fluid in the cranial vault of a decompensated patient may initiate herniation.
   b) the infused flush solution is under too much pressure.
   c) ICP may be greater than 300 mm Hg.
   d) of high infection risk.

9. Frequent complications secondary to ICP monitoring are

   a) high infection rates.
   b) seldom seen.
   c) hemorrhage.
   d) air emboli.

10. Advantages of the intraventricular techniques include

   a) intact dura.
   b) cerebrum not invaded.
   c) the ability to drain CSF and do volume pressure responses.
   d) the suitability for use in all neurosurgical patients.

11. Plateau waves, also known as "A" waves

   a) may indicate decreased intracranial compliance.
   b) are a preterminal sign.
   c) usually have a duration of less than 5 minutes.
   d) have no clinical significance.

12. ICP monitoring

   a) reduces ICP.
   b) should be initiated as quickly as possible after the clinical onset of signs and symptoms of increased intracranial pressure.
   c) is crucial in the diagnosis and management of the patient who has or may have increased intracranial pressure.
   d) is associated with an infection rate of approximately 18%.

Invasive Neurologic Assessment Techniques

ANSWERS TO STUDY QUESTIONS

1. b
2. d
3. c
4. b
5. a
6. c
7. d
8. a
9. b
10. c
11. a
12. c

Hypothermia

STUDY QUESTIONS

What is the physiological rationale and what principles of nursing care would you apply based on each of the following facts?

1. Hemoconcentration results from hypothermia.

2. Shivering is the body's initial compensatory response to cold.

3. Drugs tend to have an accumulative effect in the hypothermic patient.

4. Respiratory acidosis can result from hypothermia.

5. "Rewarming" shock can occur when hypothermia is terminated.

6. Fat necrosis is a potential occurrence when hypothermia is used.

7. In the first 15 minutes of hypothermia, all vital signs increase (blood pressure, pulse, repiration, temperature).

8. Temperature tends to continue to drift downward after the cooling blanket is turned off.

Hypothermia

ANSWERS TO STUDY QUESTIONS

1. In hypothermia, water shifts from the intravascular space to the interstitial and intracellular spaces. Sodium moves into the cell in exchange for potassium, taking water with it. The result is hemoconcentration. Nursing measures such as frequent change of body position and passive range of motion exercises are aimed at reducing embolic phenomena.
2. Shivering is a compensatory response to maintain body heat. This increased activity leads to greater oxygen consumption and, if prolonged, can result in hypoglycemia. Nursing assessment must consider these possibilities. Drug therapy (chlorpromazine [Thorazine] or promethazine

[Phenergan]) may be indicated to reduce the shivering response if it does not subside when the vasocontrictor effect is broken.

3. Drugs given subcutaneously or intramuscularly tend to accumulate in the hypothermic patient due to decreased peripheral perfusion. Decreased enzyme activity also results in slower chemical reactions. Drugs are best given intravenously or orally (by means of nasogastric tube if necessary). If intra-muscular is the recommended route, the drug should be injected *deep* into the muscle and vigilance maintained for accumulative effects during the rewarming phase.

4. Depressed ventilation during hypothermia can result in an accumulation of carbon dioxide. Assisted ventilation (respirator use) may be necessary.

5. With rapid rewarming, massive dilation of peripheral vessels occurs, resulting in decreased venous return and decreased cardiac output. When the periphery is warmed before the heart, the cool heart often cannot handle the increased peripheral demands. Rewarming is best accomplished naturally using blankets and avoiding direct heat.

6. Prolonged exposure to cold and a diminished circulation can lead to crystal formation in cellular fluid elements. Necrosis and cellular death follow. Nursing measures should be aimed at increasing circulation and preventing prolonged exposure of any body surface area to the cold source. A coating of lotion and talcum powder affords some protection to the skin.

7. In the first 15 minutes of hypothermia, shivering increases metabolic activity and all body requirements. Temperature rise reflects this increased activity and heat production. The initial vasoconstrictor response increases venous return and cardiac output, and pulse and blood pressure rise accordingly. the respiratory rate increases in response to the additional metabolic requirements for oxygen and elimination of carbon dioxide. These changes in vital signs must be interpreted in conjunction with the nurse's knowledge of the physiology of hypothermia and her total assessment of the patient.

8. Cold blood from the periphery continues to circulate and cool the body core. This process can continue to lower body temperature one to two degrees after the cooling mattress is turned off. Therefore, cooling should be discontinued before the desired temperature is reached to allow for drift downward.

Spinal Cord Injury

STUDY QUESTIONS

1. The clinical signs of hyper-reflexia include which of the following:

    a) Tachycardia   **d)** Sweating
    b) Headache   **e)** Hypertension
    c) Hypotension   **f)** Rhinorrhea

    1. a, b, e
    2. a, b, d, f
    3. b, d, f
    4. b, d, e, f
    5. c, d, f

2. Which of the following statements are true about a spinal cord contusion?

    a) A contusion usually involves some degree of anatomic interruption of cord function only.
    b) A contusion usually involves some degree of physiological interruption of cord function only.
    c) A contusion usually involves some degree of anatomic and physiological interruption of cord function.
    d) A contusion usually results in ecchymosis and swelling secondary to cord compression.
    e) A contusion usually does not imply a permanent neurologic deficit.

    1. a, d
    2. b, d, e
    3. c, d
    4. c, d, e
    5. b, e

3. From which spinal segments does the nerve supply to the bladder arise?

    a) L2 and 3 and S2, 3, and 4
    b) L3 and 4 and S1, 2, and 3
    c) L1 and 2 and S1 and 2

4. Which statements are true of a patient with an acute C 5-segment cord injury?

    a) Function of the diaphragm is impaired in the acute stage.
    b) There is intestinal paralysis.
    c) The upper extremities are outwardly rotated.
    d) The shoulders are elevated.

    1. a, b, c
    2. b, c, d
    3. a, c, d

    4. a, b, d
    5. a, b, c, d
5. Which of the following would most likely describe a patient in spinal shock as he would appear in the emergency room?
    a) pink, warm, dry skin, vasodilatation
    b) pale, cool, wet skin, vasoconstriction
6. At what level of quadriplegia can a patient usually be ventilator independent?

7. At what level of quadriplegia does a patient have the potential for independent living, without attendant care?

8. Is the orthopedic level of injury the same as the neurologic level of injury?

9. Is rectal tone by itself an indication of an incomplete cord injury?

10. Is spinal shock seen with complete spinal cord injuries or with incomplete injuries?

11. How long does it take for miscroscopic tissue changes to occur due to pressure on the skin?

12. What level of the spinal cord is responsible for psychogenic erection in males?

13. Name several conditions that could trigger an episode of autonomic dysreflexia.

Spinal Cord Injury

ANSWERS TO STUDY QUESTIONS

1. 4) b, d, e, f
2. 3) c, d
3. a
4. 5) a, b, c, d
5. a
6. C5
7. C7
8. No, not necessarily. They may be the same with a complete cord lesion but may be different with an incomplete lesion.
9. No. Rectal tone by itself, without the criterion of voluntary perianal muscle contraction or rectal sensation, is not evidence of an incomplete injury. Some rectal tone may be accounted for by local reflexes.
10. It can be seen with either.
11. Local tissue ischemia can occur in less than 30 minutes.
12. T11 to L2.
13. Bladder distention, bowel impaction, decubiti

Brain Injury

STUDY QUESTIONS

1. The neurophysiology of respiration includes:
   a) The motor strip of the cerebral cortex
   b) The medulla oblongata in the brain stem
   c) The cranial nerves IX and X
   d) The cervical and thoracic spinal nerves
   e) a, b, c,
   f) b, c, d,
   g) All of the above

2. A respiratory pattern change may indicate a further expanding lesion in the cerebral hemispheres as well as in the midbrain.

   TRUE   FALSE

3. In a patient with traumatic brain injury, the presence of Cheyne-Stokes respiration indicates the trauma was directly to the midbrain.

   TRUE   FALSE

4. Most brain-injured patients have a flaccid bladder and would retain urine without a Foley catheter in place.

   TRUE   FALSE

5. The actual mechanism of evacuating the bowel is basically a reflex activity at the spinal cord level.

   TRUE   FALSE

6. In the brain stem-injured patient, bed positioning with trunk rotation and flexion of lower extremities will help relax abnormal muscle tone and posturing.

   TRUE   FALSE

7. Positioning a brain stem-injured patient supine instead of side lying will decrease opisthotonic posturing.

   TRUE   FALSE

8. Swallowing is a complex reflex that can occur below the level of consciousness.

   TRUE   FALSE

9. A patient must be able to follow simple verbal directions before oral intake is initiated.

TRUE   FALSE

10. A large tracheostomy tube can interfere with swallowing function.

TRUE   FALSE

11. Tap water is a good choice for the first trial at oral intake.

TRUE   FALSE

12. The best position for feeding is to have the patient flat in bed.

TRUE   FALSE

13. Many patients with swallowing dysfunction have greater difficulty with liquids than with solids.

TRUE   FALSE

14. On a long-term basis, a gastrostomy tube is preferred over a nasogastric tube for patients unable to maintain total oral intake.

TRUE   FALSE

15. Oral intake should be initiated as soon after onset as possible, even if the patient has acute medical problems.

TRUE   FALSE

16. Why are sedatives not generally prescribed for agitated behavior displayed by the person with a head injury?

17. Why is it important to interrupt inappropriate emotional behavior in the brain-injured patient with affective lability?

Brain Injury

ANSWERS TO STUDY QUESTIONS

1. f) b, c, d
2. True
3. False
4. False
5. True
6. True
7. False
8. True
9. False
10. True
11. False
12. False
13. True
14. True
15. False
16. The level of consciousness (LOC) is the most reliable index for the determination of neurologic status. Vital signs often do not reflect a change in neurologic condition, while a subtle alteration in the patient's LOC should alert the nurse of changing status. Sedation would alter this index, masking what could be important cues to a neurologic crisis.
17. Such behavior is perpetual, consuming the patient's energy and interfering with the establishment of normal behavioral responses. Continuous crying or laughing should be terminated to allow the patient to gain control and to focus on appropriate behavior.

Cerebrovascular Disease

STUDY QUESTIONS

1. Following a stroke, which type of aphasia may involve slow, nonfluent speech; poor articulation; awareness of the deficit; and understanding of written and verbal speech?
   a) Expressive aphasia
   b) Receptive aphasia
   c) Global aphasia
2. With which cerebrovascular problem may a unilateral headache be the chief initial complaint?
   a) Stroke
   b) Arteriovenous malformation
   c) Hydrocephalus
3. Which cerebrovascular problem is due to a defect in the smooth muscle layer of an artery, allowing the endothelial lining to bulge through?
   a) AVM
   b) Stroke
   c) Aneurysm
4. Hemorrhage from an aneurysm most often occurs in which space in the brain?
   a) Subdural space
   b) Epidural space
   c) Subarachnoid space
5. If a patient complains of a "noise in the head," which of the following is most likely the problem?
   a) An aneurysm
   b) An AVM
   c) A stroke
   d) A psychosis
6. Photophobia, blurred vision, fever, irritability, nuchal rigidity, and positive Kernig's sign may be indicative of which of the following conditions?
   a) An intracerebral hemorrhage
   b) Meningitis or subarachnoid hemorrhage
   c) Hydrocephalus
   d) Vasospasm
   e) Ischemia or infarction

7. Which of the following conditions might be a complication of having blood in the subarachnoid space?
    1) Hydrocephalus
    2) Dysrhythmias
    3) Aphasia
    4) Hemiplegia
    5) Cranial nerve defect
        a) 4, 5
        b) 3, 4
        c) 1, 4
        d) 1, 2
        e) 2, 3

8. Which criteria describe a Grade III aneurysm?
    a) Alert, mild to severe headache, nuchal rigidity, minimal neurological deficit
    b) Deep coma, decerebrate rigidity, moribund appearance
    c) Drowsy or confused, nuchal rigidity, may have mild focal deficits
    d) Asymptomatic, alert with minimal headache, slight nuchal rigidity, no neurological deficit

9. Which type(s) of stroke typically present suddenly and progress rapidly over minutes or hours, with little or no prior warning?
    a) Hemorrhagic stroke
    b) Embolic stroke
    c) Thrombotic stroke
    d) Embolic and hemorrhagic stroke
    e) Embolic and thrombotic stroke

10. Which statement best describes an apraxia?
    a) An inability to identify the environment by means of the senses
    b) An inability to understand the written word
    c) Impairment of comprehension of the spoken word
    d) Loss of ability to use objects correctly

Cerebrovascular Disease

ANSWERS TO STUDY QUESTIONS

1. a
2. b
3. c
4. c
5. a
6. b
7. d
8. c
9. d
10. d

Seizure Disorders

STUDY QUESTIONS

1. Which class of seizures may be manifested by visual, auditory, or olfactory hallucinations or a visceral sensation prior to the seizure?
   a) Complex partial seizures
   b) Simple partial seizures
   c) Absence seizures
2. Which is the most serious and most common type of status epilepticus?
   a) Absence status
   b) Partial motor status
   c) Generalized tonic-clonic status
3. What percent of patients with status epilepticus can be controlled on a long-term basis with phenytoin?
   a) 30%
   b) 50%
   c) 80%
4. Patients with which type of seizures may follow commands and maintain eye contact with an observer?
   a) Absence seizures
   b) Pseudoseizures
   c) Complex partial seizures
5. Which type of seizure is best described in the following example: a repetitive, usually unilateral, involuntary contraction of a specific muscle group, such as thumb flexors?
   a) Simple partial seizure
   b) Complex partial seizure
   c) Atypical absence seizure
   d) Typical absence seizure

Seizure Disorders

ANSWERS TO STUDY QUESTIONS

1. a
2. c
3. c
4. b
5. a

Management of Acute Gastrointestinal Bleeding

STUDY QUESTIONS

1. Frequent assessment of the patient who has had an upper GI bleed will indicate whether or not hypovolemic shock is imminent. What will the assessment include?

2. Which lab test is most significant in a GI bleed and why?

3. Management of a GI bleed may include several dramatic procedures. One of these is the introduction of topical thrombin into the stomach. What are two important nursing precautions that must be taken?

Management of Acute Gastrointestinal Bleeding

ANSWERS TO STUDY QUESTIONS

1. Amount and frequency
   Temperature will elevate to 101° to 102°F (38.3° to 38.9°C).
   Pulse will increase to maintain adequate blood pressure.
   Respiration will increase to maintain adequate gas exchange.
   Blood pressure will drop.
   Urine output will decrease below 30 ml/hour.
   Skin will be wet from perspiration and later also cool.
   Muscular status will be characterized by weakness.
   Mental status will display anxiety.
   Bowel sounds will be hyperactive.
2. The BUN is most significant in a GI bleed. It is an excellent way to follow a bleed because it will remain elevated until approximately 12 hours after cessation of bleeding. As blood flow is decreased to the liver and kidneys and decomposed blood is absorbed from the intestines, the blood urea level will rise.
3. Aspirate stomach contents first. Thrombin must come in contact with the bleeding site. Neutralize stomach acids with a buffer solution. Stomach acids are detrimental to the treatment.

Hepatic Failure and Hyperalimentation

STUDY QUESTIONS

1. Two patients have liver disease—one has the diagnosis of infectious hepatitis while the other has the diagnosis of type B hepatitis. Even though they both have hepatitis, what makes their diseases different?

2. Since there is very little that can be done therapeutically to assist the liver's incredible natural healing process, patients with liver failure require constant and expert nursing care. Why?

3. A patient with hepatic failure may have hepatic encephalopathy, too. What are its symptoms, and what is the major treatment?

4. List three that are important for determining liver dysfunction and what the results will indicate.

5. What are the specific observations for persons on hyperalimentation?

6. What is the preferred route for hyperalimentation? Why?

Hepatic Failure and Hyperalimentation

ANSWERS TO STUDY QUESTIONS

1. Infectious hepatitis is a viral infection—type A. Lab work shows high transaminase levels and rising serum hepatitis A antibody (anti HAV). It is transmitted through the oral-fecal route, and the incidence is higher in low socioeconomic regions. Generally, persons are no longer infectious when they present with symptoms (*i.e.,* malaise, weakness, headache, nausea). Course runs 1 to 3 months and usually ends with complete recovery.

   Type B hepatitis is also a viral infection, but of type B rather than type A. Lab work shows elevated transaminase levels and elevated HBSAG. It is transmitted through body secretions and the parenteral route. If patients improve, their serum levels drop. If patients become chronic, they are also active with elevated levels of HBSAG and continue to be infectious to others. They may have liver impairment. A decreased surface antigen titer usually has a counterpart of elevating antibody to SAG. This can lead to an immune complex disease. If E antigen levels are high, the patients are probably infectious to others because they most likely have active liver disease.

2. The liver and the functions it performs are essential to life. Therefore, since it cannot adequately carry out these functions and needs to be rested while it is healing itself, medical and nursing staff can assist the body by:

Maintaining body functions not impaired by the disease (*e.g.,* respirations)

Intervening to maintain specific functions (*e.g.,* fluid balance)

Taking over functions in which failure may be complete (*e.g.,* replacement of clotting factors)

Preventing complications (*e.g.,* aspiration pneumonia, decubitus ulcers, arrhythmias)

3. Clinically, the patient may either be in a stupor, have a quiet delirium and then progress to profound coma, or he may be very agitated and difficult to manage. A hyperventilation syndrome with respiratory alkalosis also is often present.

When the liver is unable to perform its detoxification of ammonia, therapy is focused on the GI tract. This includes protein-free diet, administration of strong cathartics to cleanse, and nonabsorbable antibiotics to sterilize the bowel. These three therapies reduce the ammonia significantly.

4. *Protein studies:* The serum proteins will be depressed or the ratio of various proteins to one another will be altered.

Prothrombin time: A prolonged prothrombin time indicates severe liver loss.

Enzyme studies: SGPT is the specific enzyme, and increased amount is indicative of liver cell damage.

Bilirubin (direct and indirect): If the conjugated is *low* and the unconjugated is *high,* preliver block is indicated. If the conjugated is *high* and the unconjugated is *normal* or *decreased,* postliver block is indicated.

BSP: This is the most sensitive test; first to become abnormal and last to return to normal. If prolonged over 1 hour, it indicates the liver's inability to conjugate dye. Other illnesses can give false readings.

5. Serum blood levels of electrolytes and glucose

Fractional urine testing

Maintaining constant infusion rate

Maintaining inflammation-free infusion route

6. The subclavian vein is preferred for the following reasons: The vessel is large, and the greater blood volume dilutes the solution so that irritation to the vessel wall is diminished; the incidence of infection is lessened in this area; and it gives the patient greater freedom of movement.

Diabetic Emergencies

STUDY QUESTIONS

1. A 55-year-old man without previous known illnesses is found comatose in his apartment and brought to the hospital; the available evidence suggests he has been comatose for several days. The laboratory reports that the initial urinalysis is negative except for "large" ketonuria.
    a) What does the finding of ketonuria mean in this patient?
    b) How do you know?
    c) Explain the mechanism of his ketonuria.

2. Characterize and contrast the usual histories of onset for diabetic ketoacidosis *vs.* insulin-induced hypoglycemia.

3. Outline four key instructions to insulin-dependent diabetic patients that help to prevent episodes of ketoacidosis.

4. a) Describe the three major pathophysiological abnormalities in diabetic ketoacidosis.

b) What findings on physical examination reflect each of these?

5. List the four phases of nutrition. Characterize each as to:
    a) Relative dependence on carbohydrate *vs.* fat as an energy supply
    b) The major source of carbohydrate in each phase
    c) Their approximate durations

6. What are the compensatory mechanisms that help to prevent rapid or excessive development of the following?
    a) Hyperglycemia
    b) Metabolic acidosis
    c) Sodium depletion
What are the metabolic penalties resulting from the operation of these compensatory mechanisms?

7. On the average, what are the losses to the body of the following constituents in an adult during the development of ketoacidosis?
    a) Sodium
    b) Water
    c) Potassium
    What fraction of each of the following body compartments do these losses represent?
    a) Extracellular fluid
    b) Intracellular fluid
    c) Total body fluid

8. List at least three primary components of therapy in diabetic ketoacidosis and their major physiological benefits.

9. Outline the major clinical and biochemical features that distinguish the characteristic patient with diabetic ketoacidosis from the one with hyperosmolar nonketotic coma.

10. You suspect an insulin-dependent patient of being in the midst of a hypoglycemic episode.
    a) What steps would be appropriate to diagnose and manage this situation?

    b) Explain and justify each step.

Diabetic Emergencies

ANSWERS TO STUDY QUESTIONS

1. a) The ketonuria in this patient represents starvation ketosis rather than diabetic ketoacidosis.

b) Glycosuria is the hallmark of uncontrolled diabetes, generally preceding the development of ketonuria as diabetic control worsens. The absence of glycosuria essentially rules out the diagnosis of diabetic ketoacidosis.

c) The patient's comatose state, from whatever cause, prevented him from eating, allowing him to develop starvation ketosis. "Large" ketonuria takes 2 to 3 days to develop during starvation; the timing is thus correct. Starvation ketosis reflects the rapid, partial oxidation of free fatty acids to ketones in the liver as the body switches over from the carbohydrate economy of the fed state to the fat economy of fasting.

2. Typical Onset of Diabetic Ketoacidosis and Hypoglycemia

	Diabetic ketoacidosis	*Hypoglycemia*
Duration of onset	Hours–days	Minutes
CNS symptoms	Gradually increasing lethargy, stupor	Blurry vision, incoordination, trouble thinking clearly, personality changes
Systemic symptoms	Thirst, urination, nausea, vomiting	Tremor, sweating, tachycardia (sometimes)
Urine tests	Strongly positive for sugar, acetone	May be positive or negative for sugar

3. If an acute, intercurrent illness develops, the following instructions should be followed:

a) Take at least some insulin, even if not eating or if vomiting. A good general rule is to reduce the morning dose of intermediate-acting insulin (*e.g.,* NPH or lente) to one-half the usual; short-acting insulin may or may not be omitted.

b) Call your physician or nurse as soon as you can.

c) Test your urine every 4 to 6 hours for sugar and acetone.

d) If urine sugars remain high, take small doses of supplemental short-acting insulin (regular or semi-lente) or a second reduced dose of intermediate insulin, according to a plan worked out with the nurse or physician.

4. a) 1) Hyperglycemia

2) Salt and water (volume) depletion

3) Ketosis and acidosis

b) 1) *Hyperglycemia:* stupor or coma, thirst, polyuria

2) *Salt and water (volume) depletion:* decreased tissue turgor, dry mucosae, hypotension or shock, tachycardia

3) *Ketosis and acidosis:* fruity "acetone" breath, Kussmaul (deep or rapid) respirations

5. Fed state

a) Largely carbohydrate for energy

b) Carbohydrate coming from gut lumen

c) From onset of meal to about 3 to 4 hours later, when all nutrients absorbed from the gut

Postabsorptive state
a) Progressive switch to fat for energy, roughly 80% dependence on fat by end of this period
b) Carbohydrate is derived from breakdown of liver glycogen
c) From about 4 to 15 hours since starting the last meal

Short fasting
a) Complete switch to fat for energy, except for those tissues with obligatory dependence on carbohydrate: brain, red cells, and so forth
b) Carbohydrate made in liver (gluconeogenesis) from peripheral supplies of lactate, glycerol, amino acids; gluconeogenic rate is maximal at approximately 3 days
c) From about 15 hours to 3 weeks after starting last meal

Prolonged fasting
a) Continued maximal fat oxidation by peripheral tissues, both long-chain free fatty acids and ketone bodies serving as energy sources; ketone bodies now supply significant portion (about 60%) of brain energy
b) Continuing gluconeogenesis but at about one-third the maximal rate
c) From 3 weeks onward

6. Compensatory mechanisms for:
   a) Hyperglycemia
   1) *Glycosuria:* glucose loss in urine drains off glucose from the extracellular fluid. Unfortunately, water and salts are swept out of the body along with glucose (osmotic diuresis), producing volume depletion.
   2) *Shift of water from cells to extracellular fluid:* this water dilutes the glucose. Price paid is intracellular dehydration. Water shifts rapidly back into cells when glucose level is lowered, which can aggravate volume depletion.
   b) Metabolic acidosis
   1) *Hyperventilation:* Keeps carbonic acid (H_2CO_3) level low, protects pH of body fluid.
   2) *Dissipation of bicarbonate buffer:* Absorbs hydrogen ion, protects pH. However, as bicarbonate stores drop lower, buffering is less efficient, hyperventilation must be faster and faster to maintain pH. Ability to compensate is progressively lost, and fatal acidosis can result.
   c) Sodium depletion
   1) *Decreasing glomerular filtration (GFR):* As salt and water (volume) are lost, GFR decreases: less sodium can escape through kidneys. Decreasing GFR permits less glucose escape through kidneys, however, allowing hyperglycemia to become extreme.
   2) *Increasing aldosterone secretion:* Occurs in response to any volume loss, causes reabsorption of sodium from renal tubules back into blood, protecting sodium stores. Potassium loss is aggravated, however, since the sodium is reabsorbed in exchange for potassium excreted.

7. *Average* net losses in an adult presenting in diabetic ketoacidosis are:
   a) Sodium: about 420 mEq
   b) Water: about 6 to 7 liters
   c) Potassium: about 300 mEq

Fractional losses from various body compartments represented by loss of these quantities of solute and water are:
   a) Extracellular fluid: about 20%
   b) Intracellular water: about 11%
   c) Total body water: 15%

8. *Saline:* Both Na^+ and water are of major importance for reexpanding intravascular and extracellular volume. This reexpansion, in turn, improves blood pressure, tissue perfusion, glomerular filtration, and ultimately permits reduction in blood sugar through rapid renal glucose loss and dilution.

Insulin: Insulin shuts off the supply of ketones at its source by reducing fatty acid release from adipose tissue; similarly, release of gluconeogenic precursors (lactate, glycerol, and alanine) from peripheral tissues is shut down. Insulin also slows the rate of gluconeogenesis and ketogenesis within the liver by a direct action on hepatic cells. Blood glucose and ketone levels are thereby permitted to fall.

Bicarbonate: In severely acidotic patients (bicarbonate levels of approximately 8 mEq/liter or below), buffering capacity is pushed almost to its limit; hence, administration of intravenous bicarbonate to raise the level above 10 to 12 mEq/liter may be viewed as important, sometimes lifesaving therapy.

Potassium and phosphate: Body potassium stores are depleted in all ketoacidotic patients. Whatever the circulating potassium level is on admission, it almost invariably falls in response to the direct effects of all of the above maneuvers (*i.e.,* saline, insulin, and bicarbonate administration). Potassium administration intravenously therefore becomes important, particularly in the later phases of therapy, to keep serum levels from falling to dangerously low levels and to help restore intracellular stores.

Intracellular phosphate is also depleted; when this happens to red blood cells, oxygen is not released normally to tissues. Phosphate therapy helps to reverse these depletion effects.

9. Clinical and Biochemical Characteristics of Diabetic Ketoacidosis and Hyperosmolar Nonketotic Coma

	Diabetic ketoacidosis	*Hyperosmolar nonketotic coma*
Age	Tend to be younger patients	Generally elderly
Water depletion and hyperosmolarity	Mild–severe	Usually extreme
CNS status	Lethargy–coma	Usually comatose; focal seizures may occur
Hyperglycemia	Moderate–high (~250–1000)	Usually very high levels (>600 mg/dl, by definition)
Ketosis/acidosis	Serum ketones positive; bicarbonate depressed	Serum ketones negative; bicarbonate normal
Outcome	Usually recover	Mortality rate ~25%–50%
Underlying diabetes	Severe, insulin-dependent	Mild, non-insulin-dependent

10. **a)** **1)** If equipment is available, immediately draw blood by venipuncture for sugar determination, or measure finger-tip blood sugar with reagent strip; then administer sweetened juice or any other rapidly available form of glucose by mouth. If more than one other person is present, these two actions can be carried out almost simultaneously, thus losing the least amount of time before treatment.

2) If no blood sugar measurement is possible, give oral glucose directly, without hesitating. If the patient is too lethargic or uncooperative to take glucose by mouth, give 25 to 50 ml of 50% D/W intravenously. If IV glucose is unavailable or if a vein is not accessible, 1 mg of glucose may be given intramuscularly or subcutaneously, or 0.5 to 1.0 ml of 1 : 1000 epinephrine may be given subcutaneously.

3) Observe the patient carefully for at least 10 to 15 minutes to be sure full recovery of normal mental status has occurred. If recovery is only partial, more glucose can always be given.

4) Try to establish the reason(s) for occurrence of hypoglycemia at this particular time, and counsel adjustments in regimen to prevent reoccurrences.

b) **1)** Although in situations in which the diagnosis is completely obvious (*e.g.,* a younger, insulin-dependent diabetic who becomes progressively confused, begins to sweat, etc.) blood sugar determination may be superfluous, in many patients the diagnosis is less than clear initially. Moreover, the initial response to glucose is often equivocal; both for medical and legal reasons, therefore, documentation of hypoglycemia may be extremely important. Sampling blood for sugar level *before* significant glucose has had time to enter the circulation is often desirable.

2) Rapid treatment of hypoglycemia is generally desirable: the symptoms are, at best, unpleasant; at worst, recurrent or prolonged hypoglycemia destroys brain cells. Twenty-five to 50 ml of 50% dextrose solution provides 12.5 to 25.0 g of glucose, sufficient to raise the circulating glucose level by at least 100 to 200 mg/dl. Both glucagon and epinephrine force the liver to break down glycogen to free glucose, releasing it then into the bloodstream; they are therefore effective without needing to supply glucose from external sources.

3) Clinical response to treatment, particularly mental state, is an important piece of evidence in management of hypoglycemia. The recovery should be *rapid* (less than 10 to 15 min) and *complete* if enough glucose has been given. If it is not, the diagnosis may be in error, or the glucose given may not have been enough or, as in the presence of gastric atony, may not have reached the circulation; or finally, the hypoglycemia may have been prolonged, preventing the brain from making an immediate recovery.

4) Many, indeed most, hypoglycemic episodes in diabetic patients should be *preventable*. It is not enough, therefore, just to treat the episode successfully: every effort should be made to determine the chain of events that permitted it to happen and changes should be made as required.

Burns

STUDY QUESTIONS

1. Name the three phases of recovery following burn injury, and list the major problem associated with each.

2. Describe each of the three categories of burn depth in terms of the symptoms characteristic of each.

3. When a severely burned patient is first received in the Emergency Department, what life-saving measures must be instituted before attention is focused on the burn wound?

4. What are the major respiratory problems which may result from a severe burn?

5. List five factors which determine the severity of a burn.

6. Write nursing diagnosis, patient outcomes, and goals of nursing care for the patient in the critical care unit.

7. Why are large quantities of intravenous fluids administered immediately post burn?

8. What are the leading causes of death among burn victims? Discuss preventive measures for each.

9. Briefly describe the various methods of treating a burn wound.

10. List and briefly describe the four (4) most common personality variants which occur following burn injury. Discuss appropriate nursing intervention for each.

11. Discuss metabolic-dietary needs and associated problems in reference to the extensively burned person.

12. Briefly explain why rehabilitation measures begin in the CCU.

13. How might you "be with" the burned person so that he can cope with his emotions and fears?

14. Discuss important aspects of pain management for the burn victim.

BURNS

ANSWERS TO STUDY QUESTIONS

1. The three phases of recovery following burn injury and major problems associated with each are as follows:
   EMERGENT PERIOD: Inhalation injury, airway obstruction, decreased tissue perfusion
   ACUTE PHASE: septicemia, pneumonia
   REHABILITATION: nutrition, scarring, and contractures
2. The three categories of burn depth and characteristics of each are:
   PARTIAL-THICKNESS (FIRST DEGREE): pinkish-red, blanches from pressure, painful, and later itches and heals spontaneously.

DEEPER PARTIAL-THICKNESS (SECOND DEGREE): pinkish-red, painful blisters, and edema. If adequate epithelial cells are present, healing will be spontaneous. If the wound converts to a full-thickness wound, grafts will be necessary.

FULL-THICKNESS (THIRD DEGREE TO FOURTH DEGREE): red, white, brown, or black. Red areas do not blanch. Red streaks, painless, sunken appearance.

3. Stop the burning process:
Maintain adequate ventilation
Maintain hemodynamic stability
Assess the burn wound
Institute infection control
Institute pain control

4. Major respiratory problems are inhalation injury, which may result in upper or lower airway obstruction, and bronchopneumonia.

5. The severity of the burn wound is determined by:
The size of the area in comparison to total body surface
Depth of the burn
Location of the burn
Age of the patient
Concomitant injury or illness

6. Two major nursing diagnoses, patient outcomes, and goals of nursing care for the patient in the critical care unit include:
ND 1: Fluid volume deficit due to plasma loss, fluid shift, third spacing
PO 1: The patient will experience fluid and electrolyte balance.
GOAL: To establish and maintain adequate fluid-electrolyte balance through fluid resuscitation therapy
ND 2: Decreased tissue perfusion due to edema, thrombosis and eschar formation
PO 2: The patient will experience adequate tissue perfusion to all body parts.
GOALS: To establish and maintain tissue perfusion through fluid resuscitation therapy
To prevent edema and ischemia of wound area
To monitor tissue perfusion

7. Large quantities of intravenous fluids are administered to prevent hypovolemic shock.
Fluid shift and loss are too quick for the body's mechanisms to maintain its equilibrium.
After 48 hours, capillaries will have sealed, and fluid loss will decrease, reversing the fluid shift.

8. The leading causes of death are septicemia and pneumonia. Infection control includes such things as the use of sterile sheets and blankets; topical antibacterial therapy; and penicillin given prophylactically for 5 days following the burn for prevention of overwhelming streptococcal infection. Nursing measures to prevent pneumonia include coughing, deep breathing, and repositioning every 1 to 2 hours as well as periodic suctioning and chest physiotherapy. Respiratory parameters should be closely monitored so that signs of complications can be detected early.

9. Burn wounds may be treated by:
OPEN WOUNDS: left open to air
HYDROTHERAPY: to clean and debride wounds or apply medication
SEMI-OPEN WOUNDS: thin layers of cream alone or in combination with a single layer of gauze
OCCLUSIVE DRESSINGS: fine mesh gauze applied directly to the wound and covered with dry fluffy gauze for absorption
WET DRESSINGS: gauze saturated with saline or silver nitrate 0.5% applied directly to the wound and covered with dry dressings
BIOLOGICAL DRESSINGS: Grafts of animal skin or man-made films are temporary coverings. Autografts of person's own skin are permanent.

ANTIMICROBIAL MEDICATIONS: silver sulfadiazine 1% (Silvadine) sulfamylon acetate 10%
ENZYMATIC DEBRIDEMENT: Travase, Elase

10. The four most common personality variants following burn injury are:

DEPRESSION: Patient may withdraw. Nurse should clarify expectations to communicate hope.

REGRESSION: Patient is unable to cope on an adult level. Nurse must accept patient's inability to cope, devise ways to assist patient to cope, and return control by permitting choices in care.

PARANOIA: Patient transfers fears to a specific caregiver. Staff member may need to be reassigned.

SCHIZOPHRENIA: Exhaustion and pain medications may lead to confusion, hallucinations, and combativeness. This usually disappears by time of discharge.

11. A severely burned person has increased metabolic rate requiring a high caloric diet to meet his energy demand—50 to 80 calories per kg of body weight, with 2 g to 3 g of protein. Supplementary vitamins and iron may be necessary. Usually the person has a conflict. On the one hand, he does not feel hungry. As a matter of fact, he feels full and may have diarrhea. On the other hand, he needs to consume a high protein/carbohydrate diet.

12. Rehabilitation measures must be started immediately to prevent scarring and contractures. The two most important ones are range of motion exercises and splinting extremities in functional positions. Later, the person may be fitted with a continuous pressure garment to control scar formation.

13. From all of the above, you know that the nurse who works with a burn patient must be a "human doer." Yet, equally as important, she must also be a "human being." An honest, compassionate team and individual approach will help the person accept his own humanness and cope with his many and overwhelming feelings. An example might be as follows:

The patient asks if "it looks ugly." It is not entirely truthful to answer, "No, it does not. It is very clean and filling-in nicely." Too often that is the answer to the question, "How does it look?" His question is deeper and cannot be so quickly answered. The nurse needs to be truthful with the person and not dodge his questions so artfully. Trust is an essential ingredient in the relationship.

14. Coverage of the wound may decrease air currents and decrease pain.

Calm, knowledgeable care will reduce anxiety.

Restlessness may indicate hypoxia.

Small IV doses of narcotics are most effective. IM administration should be avoided.

The stability of the staff and incorporation of the family into care are important for providing emotional support.

Effects of the Critical Care Unit on the Nurse

STUDY QUESTIONS

1. Name five of the major stresses that critical care nurses experience consistently in their work.

2. Define coping. What are the two main components of coping? In what mental structure does coping primarily occur?

3. Name three defense mechanisms that many CCU nurses develop as a response to the stress of their work.

4. Describe the differences found in studies of intensive and nonintensive care nurses with regard to power, detachment, and anxiety.

5. Describe the qualities of a selfless person.

6. Name three causes of burnout.

7. Name three characteristics of each of the following behaviors:
   a) Passive behavior

   b) Aggressive behavior

   c) Assertive behavior

8. Name four basic rights of women in the health care professions.

9. Define "professional distancing."

10. What are the three sources of conflict that nurses experience in the CCU?

11. Name four ways in which CCU nurses can relieve some of the stress of working in the critical care environment.

12. Name five ways in which hospital administrations can decrease the stress on CCU nurses (and at the same time decrease costly nursing turnover).

DISCUSSION TOPICS

As an adjunct to the study questions, you may find it helpful to further explore the issues raised in this chapter in a group setting. The leadership role should be filled by someone trained in group dynamics. Adequate time should be allowed for discussion of each topic.

1. Take about 5 minutes and list the qualities you expect of yourself as a nurse. Use oneword adjective descriptions. Compare your self-expectations with those of the other group members. Are these expectations reasonable? Justify your reasoning.

2. In this exercise the group leader should read the following statements to the group. Discussion should follow each statement.

   What is guilt? What does guilt feel like?

   Read the following: Very small children do not feel guilt. They acquire it as they are socialized by their parents and society at large. Is it possible that nurses acquire more guilt feelings in the process of becoming nurses? If so, how?

   How does guilt affect the way that nurses do their jobs?

3. Write down the two leading causes of burnout in nurses. Compare the two causes you have chosen with those of the other group members. Have you identified similar stresses? Discuss your findings.

4. Nursing has been identified as the profession with the highest job turnover rate. In working to improve working conditions, is it better for nurses to help their own group within the hospital, such as critical care nurses, pediatric nurses, and so forth, or for all nurses within the hospital to work together? Why? Is it possible for a large nursing group such as the American Nurses' Association to effect changes that could decrease the turnover rate in this country? Justify your reasoning.

5. Read the five basic rights of women in the health professions aloud to the group:

   You have the right to be treated with respect.

   You have the right to a reasonable workload.

   You have the right to a reasonable wage.

   You have the right to determine your own priorities.

   You have the right to ask for what you want.

   After each right is read, ask the group to discuss their reaction to it.

   What did you *feel* as the right was being read?

   After each right has been discussed ask the following question:

   Are some of the rights more achievable than others?

   Which ones and why?

6. *Role playing:* Describe an example of a nurse's right being violated in the critical care unit. Any example can be chosen by the group. Have a group choose players to represent the various characters involved in the situation. Role play the incident three times. The person playing the nurse should demonstrate three different behaviors: passive, aggressive, and assertive. The group should discuss after each portrayal their reactions to the three different behaviors and the reactions of the other characters in the incident to the different behaviors of the nurse.

7. Discuss the personality characteristics you think would be ideal for a CCU nurse. Explain your reasons.

Effects of the Critical Care Unit on the Nurse

ANSWERS TO STUDY QUESTIONS

1. Unpredictability of the environment
   Sensory overload: sights, sounds, and so forth
   Repetitive routine
   Frequent charting
   Acute crisis situations
   Emotional outbursts of patients

Physical exertion
Working in close proximity with others

2. Coping is a combination of conscious strategies that have worked successfully in the past and unconscious defense mechanisms, in order to reduce the level of stress that a person is experiencing.

   Its main components are conscious coping strategies, stress management techniques, and so on.

   Coping primarily occurs in the ego.

3. Denial
   Repression
   Withdrawal
   Avoidance

4. Power: The CCU nurses generally felt less powerful and more controlled by their environment than non-CCU nurses.
   Detachment: The CCU nurses were more detached or experienced less of an acute awareness of their environment than non-CCU nurses.
   Anxiety: CCU nurses experience less anxiety in both new and normal situations than non-CCU nurses.

5. Devoted to the needs of others
   Needs of self are not acknowledged
   Self-motivated when a need is observed
   Remains subordinate to the dictates of an institution

6. Denial of self
   Chronic understaffing
   Increasing rate of technologic change
   Hopelessness about changes that would improve the working conditions
   Lack of resolution about the loss of patients

7. *Passive behavior:*
   Deceptive about own feelings
   Yielding
   Self-denying
   Aggressive behavior:
   Quarrelsome
   Bold
   Degrades others
   Assertive behavior:
   Open
   Honest
   Does not impinge on others' beliefs

8. You have the right to be treated with respect.
   You have the right to a reasonable workload.
   You have the right to an equitable wage.
   You have the right to determine your own priorities.
   You have the right to ask for what you want.

9. It is a "numbness' of feelings in the nurse, a lessening of reactions to difficult situations of any kind. This involves a loss of awareness of the emotional needs of patients and their families. It is a pulling away of nurses' involvement and emotional commitment to their patients.

10. Nurse-doctor relationships
    Lack of resolution of deaths of patients
    Intra-staff schisms
    Competition with other nurses

11. Engage in physical exercise after working hours.

Attend academic or other types of classes in order to develop another mental focus.

Participate in a psychiatric liaison group.

Rotate out of the CCU onto a step-down unit at specific intervals.

Assign orderlies the task of preparing deceased patients for the morgue.

Actively work at maintaining communication and group cohesiveness within unit staff (including the head nurse).

12. CCU nurses need strong moral support and respect from nursing supervisors.

Nursing administration needs to recognize the importance of a support group to CCU staff on a consistent, ongoing basis.

This support requires budgeting both time for staff members to attend meetings, so that adequate coverage is available, and financial resources for a qualified psychiatric liaison or similarly-prepared group leader.

Employ a full-time physician as permanent director of the CCU.

Implement the following policies if requested by the nursing staff:

   Allow 6 full weeks for orientation of new nursing personnel.

   Upgrade nurse-patient ratios as technologic changes advance or patient care situations become particularly acute.

   Pay CCU nurses an extra wage increment, especially when chronic understaffing occurs.

   Schedule a senior staff nurse on the day shift with a lighter patient assignment. She can assist and teach the less experienced staff.

   Implement 4-day work weeks.

Incorporate the following architectural changes into new construction or renovations:

   Allow larger space between patient beds

     or

   Build small rooms so that patients are separated from one another.

   Build nurses' lounge out of view of patients.

   Install windows in the unit.

   Install clocks within sight of patient.

   Install extra amounts of sound-deadening material.

Training and Development of Critical Care Nursing Staffs

The following section is composed of guides for persons who have accepted the position and role of staff educator. It is important that each step be taken and each guide completed. It will clarify assumptions and validate reality, avoiding many pitfalls that can occur from unrealistic expectations and false assumptions. Be patient with yourself and allow yourself the time to be thoughtful and quiet.

GUIDE 1

Directions

Everyone has work, personal, and life goals. Many times, they are never articulated. An excellent starting point is to write your own goals in the three areas listed. Perhaps at the moment, you think you haven't any. Search your thoughts. They are there!

Work	Personal	Life
My professional goals are:	My social goals are:	My life goals are:

GUIDE 2

Directions

To determine the compatibility of your goals with staff and organization, the following is offered.

Personal	Unit	Organization
Philosophy I believe:	My staff believes:	My organization believes:
	My patients believe:	
Needs I need:	Staff needs:	My organization needs:
	My patients need:	

My revised goals are:

GUIDE 3

Directions

Categorize the needs of each group into needs and wants. Validate their existence. Then you are ready to put the needs into general areas. Once this is completed, you are ready to construct objectives for each general area.

General Need Areas	Objectives
1.	1.
2.	2.
3.	3.

GUIDE 4

Directions

For each objective, list those factors that currently exist that would enhance or hinder the process for reaching it. What activities could remove the blocks, and what could support the process?

Objective: Hindrance (blocks)   Enhance

Activities to remove blocks   Activities to encourage

Objective: Hindrance (blocks)   Enhance

Activities to remove blocks   Activities to encourage

Continue on with each objective. A word of caution: some blocks may seem impossible to remove. Perhaps rewording the block will bring new ideas.

GUIDE 5

Directions

Select one objective that is important to those participating in the teaching-learning process, one that will have immediate payoff and few risks, and one that will set a positive tone for future experiences.

Objective:

Activities to reach this objective: Resources available:

Anticipated payoffs: Payoffs obtained:

Staff evaluation: Self-evaluation: